DARE
to **BARE**

DARE to **BARE**

THE COMPLETE DIET AND FITNESS PROGRAMME FOR YEAR-ROUND BODY CONFIDENCE

By the Experts from

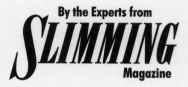

SLIMMING Magazine

Edited by Christine Michael

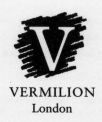

VERMILION
London

ACKNOWLEDGEMENTS

Many people have contributed to the success of *Slimming* over the years and therefore, to this book. In particular, the following have all lent their skill and knowledge to these pages:

Mary Atkinson, Felicity Bates, Patience Bulkeley, Dr John Cobb, Dr Elizabeth Evans, Dell Gibbens, Sara Gilbert, Sybil Greatbatch, Gaynor Hagan, Erika Harvey, Peter Honey, Sarah Johnson, Juliette Kellow, Jon LeBon, Sarah Litvinoff, Chris McGlaughlin, Glynis McGuinness, Libby Roberts, Kandy Shepherd, Michele Simmons, Ming Tang-Evans.

1 3 5 7 9 10 8 6 4 2

Text copyright © Slimming Magazine/Emap Elan Ltd 1998

First published in the United Kingdom in 1998 by Vermilion
an imprint of Ebury Press
Random House
20 Vauxhall Bridge Road
London SW1V 2SA

Random House Australia (Pty) Limited
18 Poland Road, Glenfield,
Auckland 10, New Zealand

Random House South Africa (Pty) Limited
Endulini, 5A Jubilee Road,
Parktown 2193, South Africa

Random House UK Limited Reg. No. 954009

A CIP catalogue record for this book is available from the British Library

ISBN: 0 09 181554 1

Printed and bound in Great Britain by
Cox & Wyman Ltd, Reading, Berkshire

Contents

Introduction:
Why Dare to Bare *is different*

Welcome to *Dare To Bare,* a different kind of diet book. Why and how is it different? The answer lies in the second part of the book's title: *The Complete Diet and Fitness Programme for Year-Round Body Confidence.* Just think for a moment of the benefits of being body-confident all year round: no more panics before holidays or parties to starve off a few pounds; no more wardrobes with 'fat clothes' and 'thin clothes'; no more guilt about bingeing or 'fattening foods'; no more making the same resolution every year to 'lose weight or else'! *Dare To Bare* is different because its promise is far more exciting and effective than 'just another diet'.

Dare To Bare starts with a huge advantage. In this book you will find the concentrated result of nearly 30 years of knowledge and experience built up in *Slimming* magazine, which was founded in 1969 by nutrition pioneer Audrey Eyton. In those days the idea of healthy eating was nothing like as popular or accepted as it is today, and *Slimming* was a world leader in making nutrition science relevant and useful for everyone.

Today, you can hardly open a newspaper or magazine or switch on the television without seeing the latest news about food health and safety or hearing a new diet guru holding forth.

As a nation, we are probably better-informed about how to eat healthily and get fit than any previous generation. Yet, ironically, even though more people are on diets and buying 'slimming foods' than ever, the worrying truth is that more people than ever are overweight and levels of obesity – where surplus weight begins to pose a real risk to health – is on the increase too.

Some pundits and pressure-groups lay the blame for this situation at the door of the diet industry itself, claiming that the very process of dieting encourages long-term weight gain and unhealthy relationships with food. Their slogan is '95 per cent of diets don't work', with the implied suggestion that any attempt to control and maintain weight is pointless and even risky.

Certainly, many of us who've tried dozens of diets, only to fall at the first hurdle or to succeed for a while and then find weight creeping back on again, might agree that 95 per cent or even 100 per cent of the diets we've tried don't work.

However, the irrefutable clinical evidence that diets *do* work is based on a very simple equation: if you consistently take in less energy (or calories) than the energy (or calories) you expend, *you will lose weight*. An equal balance of energy intake and expenditure should result in weight being maintained, but a consistent surplus of energy in over energy out will result in gradual weight gain.

As with all apparently simple truths, other factors may need to be taken into account. For example, the energy in–energy out balance can be temporarily upset by illness or by medication.

But, for the majority of basically healthy people who would like to lose some weight and keep it off, the great news is that you no longer need to worry about the 95 per cent of diets that 'don't work'. All you have to do is to find a way of reducing your energy intake and increasing your energy expenditure that *works for you*. And that's what

Dare To Bare will make it easy for you to do – and that's why *Dare To Bare* is different.

In this book you won't find a single diet that we recommend for all readers like a 'one size fits all' T-shirt. That's because at *Slimming* we have learnt that the long-term successful slimmers are those who find a pattern of eating and exercise that suits their body, their tastes and their lifestyle so that they are able to accommodate anything life throws at them, all year round. Through trial and error they discover how to carry on enjoying the foods they like best, how to cope with eating out, stressful situations and busy lives and how to fit in exercise that they enjoy. By definition, that pattern is different for everyone; it's not something you can just hand out on a diet-sheet.

So, in *Dare To Bare,* you won't find a miracle diet that you might stick to for a while but find hard to sustain or enjoy in the long term. You *will* find:

- all the tools you need to discover what will work for you
- strategies to help you defeat some of the 'dieting demons' that may have hampered your weight-loss plans in the past
- sound and sensible advice to put together your *own* formula for successful, safe slimming
- delicious calorie- and fat-controlled recipes for every season of the year
- easy exercises and suggestions on how to boost your fitness.

If you follow the *Dare To Bare* philosophy, there are no instant solutions and you may find you don't succeed in finding your winning formula immediately. This book asks you to make a commitment, but remember that anyone can go on a diet; it takes someone special to be a successful slimmer. Let *Dare To Bare* be your guide to year-round body confidence and you need never worry about dieting again!

1

What's your dieting style?

Quiz 1: Discover your diet personality

Discovering your hidden motivation could mean the difference between the success and failure of your diet. Complete the short quiz below to find out whether you are driven by the pleasure principle or the fear of failure, and to find your ideal dieting style.

Answer the following questions as honestly as you can, and remember that there are no rights or wrongs. You may fit into more than one of the categories. In this case, choose the statement that is most true to you. It's worth spending time thinking carefully about your answers, as they could help you become more aware of the way you approach slimming. What's more, they could help you make changes that will boost your motivation – and therefore your chances of success!

1 It's Monday morning. Today is the day that you promised to start a new healthy-eating and exercise programme. As you push back the bedclothes, what thoughts come to mind?
   (a) 'I look and feel so awful when I'm fat. But what if I don't achieve my goal? I'll feel even worse then.'

(b) 'What have I let myself in for? It's all going to be too much. I'm not going to be able to cope. I can't see an end to it. I'll put it off until next week.'

(c) 'What's for breakfast? I want something to eat.'

(d) 'This is the start of the new me. I'm really looking forward to reaching my target weight and enjoying a sense of achievement.'

2 If you were asked to draw a picture of yourself on a diet, which of these images would be nearest?

(a) You look fat and unhappy.

(b) Your face and body reflect pain and deprivation; you're swamped by piles of diet-sheets and weighing scales.

(c) You're enjoying a meal – a calorie-counted meal, that is.

(d) You have a smiling face, and the picture shows you in the future, maybe window-shopping for a new wardrobe of clothes.

3 Look ahead to how you imagine yourself in a couple of years time. How do you picture yourself?

(a) You'd rather not think that far ahead. You look so dreadful as you are that it would be too upsetting to think that you could still look this bad, or even worse.

(b) Still overweight, still trying to diet and still failing miserably.

(c) You've no idea. Forward thinking is not your style.

(d) Absolutely gorgeous. You will have reached your target weight and you'll be enjoying your new figure to the full.

4 You've had a hard day and you're tired and hungry, but it's not supper-time yet. You head straight for the larder or fridge when you get home. As you look at the contents, what do you say to yourself?

(a) 'I know that I ought to wait until supper, but I don't want to – I'm too hungry and fed up. Why should I keep depriving myself? I don't mind what I have as long as it fills the gap and stops me feeling so tense and miserable.'

(b) 'I know that I ought to be good, but I can't face any more dieting. I'll eat something now, and start the diet another time.'

(c) 'I'm going to choose the food that most appeals to my tastebuds, the thing that will immediately make me feel good, even if it's high in calories.'

(d) 'I have a choice. Either I can eat something nourishing and filling like some raw vegetables or a cup of soup, or I can treat myself to a small cake or a biscuit and adjust my calorie allowance later.'

5 You go to bed after a party, knowing that you have overindulged. What do you say to yourself?

(a) 'I feel dreadful and it serves me right. I'm such a pig, it's no wonder that I look so fat and frumpy.'

(b) 'That's it! I'm useless. I knew that I wouldn't be able to keep to a diet. I don't know why I even bothered to try.'

(c) 'It's typical of me. I just love food so much I can't resist it.'

(d) 'Never mind, I'm allowed the odd indulgence. I'm not going to let it interfere with my long-term goal. I've done well up until now. I'll get straight back on the diet again tomorrow.'

6 A friend suggests that you go to a new exercise class together. She offers to pick you up and take you, so there's no way of getting out of it. As you travel to the leisure centre, how do you picture yourself in the class?

(a) Hot, sticky and miserable. Your figure will look even worse in comparison with the others in the class.

(b) You just know you're going to make a fool of yourself. You can see yourself failing to keep up with the others and leaving before the class is over.

(c) You'd rather not think that far ahead. If you had to picture yourself it would probably be enjoying a cool drink in the café afterwards.

(d) Glowing with the exertion and 'feel-good' hormones. You may not be able to keep up with the others, but you're giving it your best because you'd like to start coming on a regular basis.

7 When you read stories about successful slimmers, how do they make you feel?

(a) You know exactly how the slimmers felt when they started their diet. Reading their stories highlights how dreadful you feel about yourself.

(b) Even more daunted by the whole prospect of dieting. You know that you ought to feel inspired but, to be honest, you don't think you could go through all that hard work for so long.

(c) It's a good read and you pick up some useful tips, but you don't really identify with the feelings the slimmers experience when they reach their target.

(d) If they can do it, so can you. You love reading success stories because it makes you feel excited about how you'll feel when you reach target weight.

8 You've lost half a stone. A friend notices and compliments you on your weight loss. How do you reply to her flattering words?

(a) 'I might have lost some weight but I still look pretty awful. There are rolls of fat around my stomach.'

(b) 'I don't think that I can keep it up much longer. I can't bear the thought of the next few weeks without a take-away.'

(c) 'I'm enjoying looking and feeling better.'

(d) 'I'm getting there. If you think I look better now, just wait another few months!'

9 A friend offers you a chocolate from a box. What do you say to yourself?

(a) 'I know that chocolates aren't allowed on my diet but I'd just feel too awful if I deprived myself, so I'll take one.'

(b) 'Now that I've seen these chocolates I'm going to keep longing for one. If I don't eat one I'm going to feel unsettled all day long.'

(c) 'There's no doubt in my mind. I'm going to have my favourite chocolate and enjoy it.'

(d) 'I know how pleased I'll feel with myself if I refuse, so I won't have one.'

10 Your summer holiday brochure arrives. Only two months to go now, but you haven't lost as much weight as you had hoped. What is your reaction most likely to be?

(a) Seeing the brochures makes you feel fat and fed up. You can't help thinking how ugly you'll look on holiday.

(b) You just know the holiday is going to be spoiled by your failure to lose weight, so you may as well face up to your weaknesses. You ask yourself why you can't ever seem to pull yourself together.

(c) You sit down and enjoy reading the brochures.

(d) This is just the incentive that you need to get back on course. You'll enjoy the holiday so much more if you are slim enough to look lovely in a bikini.

Look back over your answers to find out how you scored.

Mostly (a)'s

The driving force behind your behaviour tends to be avoiding anything that will cause you immediate or short-term pain in any way. You tend to act rather impulsively, usually seeing the negative side of yourself and others. You have a tendency to put yourself down, focusing on thinking how bad you look rather than on your good points. You talk to yourself in a stern voice, rather like a strict schoolteacher, and then rebel against authority.

Your dieting style

Be kinder to yourself. See yourself in a new light: rather than worrying about how you look now, think about how you'll look and feel when you are slimmer and fitter. And look beyond the pain of depriving yourself to the longer-term goal of dieting success and all the rewards that it brings.

Mostly (b)'s

You tend to foresee problems before you've even begun your diet, and try to avoid anything that will cause you pain in the long term. The thought of the actual dieting process and all the difficulties that it may entail makes you question your ability to cope. You can be easily overwhelmed by the thought of dieting, seeing it as a much bigger hardship than it really is. It's no wonder that you so often put it off until next week and then end up feeling even more daunted.

Your dieting style

Take a step-by-step approach, so that the task ahead is not so daunting. Instead of concentrating on all the hardships, think about the more positive side of dieting: how self-control will boost your self-esteem, how much more confident you will feel, and how proud you will be of yourself. Rather than wasting time longing for high-calorie foods that you can't fit into your calorie allowance, think about all the nourishing and tasty foods that you *can* eat on your diet.

Mostly (c)'s

You're an impetuous character. You live for the minute and want to enjoy life to the full. You're driven by the desire for instant pleasure. As you tuck into that slice of gateau, you savour every mouthful and don't think ahead to how you will feel when you realize that you have broken your diet.

Your dieting style
Look one step beyond your wish for immediate gratification to how your action will make you feel. If it's going to cause you pain (whether through feelings of guilt, remorse or failure), stop yourself. You need more goal orientation to help your motivation. Set small goals along the way, taking one day at a time. And think further ahead, to the lasting pleasure you will gain from achieving your target weight.

Mostly (d)'s

Your behaviour is shaped by the wish to move towards long-term pleasure. If this is your attitude, you're likely to succeed at your diet. You will take all the rigours of dieting in your stride because you know they are necessary. You talk to yourself in an encouraging way, always confident that you'll succeed. You'll take every opportunity to boost your self-motivation by looking ahead to how you will feel and look when you have achieved your goal.

Your dieting style
You're a natural! Keep up the good work.

Quiz 2: What kind of diet should you follow?

A diet is not a diet unless you can stick to it. The most important thing to ask yourself before you embark on your diet is 'will it fit into my lifestyle?'

If your place of work doesn't have cooking facilities, there is no way you will be able to stick to a diet that requires you to cook a meal every lunch-time. If you cook a large meal for your family in the evening, you may find it difficult to keep to a diet that asks you to eat your main meal at midday. The best diet for you is one that makes it easy for you to control your calorie and fat intake.

Use this questionnaire to find out what sort of diet is most suited to your lifestyle, temperament and taste.

For each question, tick or circle the statement that best describes your situation. Choose only one statement per question. Then count up how many a's you choose, how many b's and so on. The answers will show which one of five types of diet should suit you best, and will help you plan your slimming campaign.

1 Do you:
   (a) enjoy take-away and convenience foods?
   (b) like to eat wholesome family meals and make meal-times social occasions for all the family?
   (c) prefer not to eat meat or fish, or follow a lacto-vege-tarian diet?
   (d) like to eat little and often?
   (e) like to have someone to advise you what you should eat and when?

2 Do you:
   (a) often have no time to plan and prepare your meals?
   (b) think it's important to spend time preparing meals for your family?
   (c) get annoyed with diets that waste your time because they are not designed for vegetarians?
   (d) like to spend as little time in the kitchen as possible when preparing meals and snacks?
   (e) hate having to figure out options and choices on a diet?

3 Are you:
   (a) prepared to spend as much money as you need to on convenience meals while you are dieting?
   (b) concerned with getting the best possible value for money from your family shopping budget?
   (c) willing to spend money on vegetarian alternatives, whether or not you're a strict vegetarian?
   (d) willing to spend as much as you need to on a diet, rather than having to stick to a strict budget?
   (e) eager to know what you're spending each day, whether it's money or calories?

4 Which statement best describes your situation?
   (a) 'For me, breakfast comes straight out of a packet, it's never cooked.'
   (b) 'I like to ensure that my family starts the day with a good breakfast.'
   (c) 'Bacon and sausages will never appear on my breakfast menu.'
   (d) 'I enjoy a bowl of cereal for supper as much as I do for breakfast.'
   (e) 'Breakfast is not my favourite meal of the day.'

5 Do you:
   (a) avoid cooking where possible?
   (b) love cooking and trying out new recipes?
   (c) enjoy the challenge of creating delicious and varied vegetarian meals?
   (d) prefer preparing snacks to conventional meals?
   (e) prefer following set menus and recipes to having to make up your own ideas?

6 Complete this sentence: 'The main reason I find losing weight difficult is . . . '
   (a) 'I am the only person with a weight problem in my family and I need separate, no-fuss meals.'
   (b) 'I have to cook family meals every day.'
   (c) 'I am vegetarian and I worry that I'm not getting enough protein. As a result, I eat lots of cheese.'
   (d) 'I suffer from PMS and feel the need to eat frequently throughout the day.'
   (e) 'I can't stick to a diet if I have to think about it too much.'

7 Choose the statement which best describes the way you feel:
   (a) 'I don't enjoy uncooked fruit and vegetables.'
   (b) 'I like to cook my family's meals so I know exactly what goes into them.'
   (c) 'I like experimenting with beans, lentils and other non-animal proteins.'
   (d) 'I prefer snacking on fruit salad to a whole fruit.'
   (e) 'I love to eat fruit and salad vegetables every day.'

8 How would you finish this sentence? 'I find it easier to lose weight if . . . '
   (a) 'everything is pre-prepared, pre-measured and calorie-counted for me.'

(b) 'I integrate my meals with my family's.'

(c) 'I eliminate meat and fish completely from my diet.'

(d) 'I'm allowed to eat a little bit of something quick and easy whenever I feel hungry.'

(e) 'I'm told exactly what to eat and when without having to do too much work.'

How did you score?

If you scored three or more (a)'s:
You are a 'Ready-to-eat dieter'. You need to choose a diet that uses easily prepared convenience foods, as you have neither the time nor the inclination to cook or to plan and think about what you eat. Look for no-fuss, rapid routes to weight loss to keep your motivation high.

If you scored three or more (b)'s:
You are a 'Family dieter'. If you are feeding a family on a fixed budget, you must find a diet that allows for this. You will do best with a diet that allows you to cook wholesome, tasty meals that the family will enjoy and that can be fitted into your calorie or fat allowance.

If you scored three or more (c)'s:
You are a 'Vegetarian dieter'. Even if you do not think of yourself as a vegetarian, your lifestyle will probably adapt well to a meat-free diet. Follow a well-balanced eating plan to ensure you get enough of all the nutrients you need.

If you scored three or more (d)'s:
You are a 'Grazing dieter'. You like to eat little and often. Choose a diet that allows you to nibble your way through the day, to keep hunger pangs at bay and food preparation at a minimum.

If you scored three or more (e)'s:
You are a 'No-nonsense dieter'. You don't want to spend time thinking about your diet. You want to be told exactly what to eat and when. Choose an eating plan that limits your choice to straightforward calorie- or fat-controlled meals with no options or extras.

2

Defeat your dieting demons

Man does not live by bread alone, and there is certainly far more to losing weight successfully than just food and diets. Most of us these days have at least some idea of what healthy eating involves, and what we should and shouldn't eat in order to slim, but putting it all into practice can seem impossible at times. This is because human beings are more than just calorie machines, able to regulate our consumption and expenditure of energy by flicking a switch. When it comes to our attitudes and approach to slimming, each of us has our own baggage of prejudices, past experiences, fears and obstacles that can get in the way of our good intentions to eat healthily, exercise and slim. Unless we tackle our own personal dieting demons, any diet we undertake is likely to be more difficult and may even be doomed to failure.

Here we look at some of the most common dieting demons and strategies for how to defeat them. See if one or more of them strikes a chord with you.

Don't let anger make you fat

Do you ever find yourself absent-mindedly picking at food all day long while a domestic or work annoyance simmers at the back of your mind? How often have you found yourself sitting in the kitchen, a half-eaten, high-calorie snack in front of you, barely aware that you have pushed the other half down while seething about an injustice that has been done to you? If your answers to these questions are 'yes' and 'very often', you could be one of the many people who use food to help dissolve their anger.

None of us can avoid getting angry once in a while. There are, of course, people who appear not to get angry, who smile calmly whatever the situation and whatever the provocation. But many of us confuse not expressing anger (by shouting or lashing out, for example) with not feeling it. This is partly because, in our minds, showing anger is linked with aggression. Being aggressive, either verbally or physically, is not acceptable in our society. So, rather than risk people forming a bad impression of us, we purse our lips, smile, and delude ourselves into thinking that everything is fine.

What we forget is that anger is a perfectly natural, healthy, human reaction. It is nature's way of preparing us for a fight. When we're angry, our blood pressure rises, our heart beats faster, our blood sugar increases, and our muscles become more tense. If we were living in the wild and another animal came along and took the food that we had just caught, these changes would give our bodies the energy they'd need to get the food back. In our modern society we rarely need to defend ourselves physically, and unless we find a way to avoid feeling angry or to express anger when we *do* feel it, repeated bouts of anger can wear us out physically and leave us tired and stressed.

For some people, food provides the perfect way to diffuse the anger they feel. For one thing, eating causes a distraction. Many women report that overeating makes them feel numb and empty of all thoughts. They literally swallow their anger. Others use food as a way to relieve tension. The act of eating is relaxing and the boost of sugar from a carbohydrate binge can produce a 'high', along with a temporary 'don't-care' attitude. Some people say that they feel lethargic after eating a large amount of food, and while they are in this state, it is difficult to continue feeling angry or to think about expressing that anger effectively.

Take the case of Rachel, a mother of four and herself the eldest of four children.

Rachel

Her mother had always been outwardly calm and gentle, but her father was constantly on a short fuse, and Rachel often had to protect her brothers from taking a beating for a minor misdemeanour. Rachel's husband, with whom she generally got on very well, was often under stress as he worked all hours in the family restaurant. As a result, he often exploded at her and the children if they disagreed with him. In her role as peacemaker, Rachel rarely responded, but seethed inside and comforted herself with sweets from the children's 'treats' box.

When Rachel began to analyse her situation, she realized that she would have to respond to her husband's abuse by expressing her anger with him, so that he in turn would have to find an alternative way of dealing with his stress. Rachel found it difficult to express anger, because of what it had meant in her childhood, and because she thought it was not 'nice' for a woman to appear to lose control. But when she considered the disadvantages of continuing to eat to avoid confronting her feelings, she realized that in fact she had no alternative. Allowing herself to shout back at her husband gave her a new feeling of control, and freed her from the need to swallow the build-up of anger with food.

There are many different sorts of situations that can make someone angry, but there is probably one type of event that provokes you more than another. It may be a direct attack, physical or verbal, or it may be the feeling that you are the victim of an injustice. You may become angry when you see someone making an annoying mistake, or when you make one yourself. Alternatively, you may feel frustrated when something or someone blocks your way and stops you from achieving your goals. In order to express your anger more freely, or to dispel it altogether, you need to consider its cause.

Angela

Angela works in the library of a large public company and takes pride in her work, which is always competent and orderly. But the behaviour of her manager constantly annoyed her. He would 'borrow' company materials for personal use and block her requests for promotion. The fact that his work was not as good as hers compounded Angela's frustration. As a single parent, dependent on her job for money, she was frightened of upsetting her manager and felt she had no option but to continue to allow him to walk all over her. So, instead of reacting, she took refuge in a store of chocolate and crisps she kept in her desk drawer.

Feeling that she was being treated unfairly, Angela needed to deal with the situation once and for all. She knew she had to learn to be more assertive, to make her demands in such a way that her boss couldn't continue to refuse her, but her attempts to speak her mind were cramped by an overpowering fear that she might be criticized because she was too fat and a single parent. So she first had to separate her negative feelings about herself as a person from her knowledge that she was very good at her job. Soon her new-found strength at work began to help her build up her self-esteem and, as a consequence, her ability to keep to a diet.

If you suspect that anger might be contributing to your dieting lapses, keep a record of the times when you stray from your diet and note what events are happening at those times. Are you aware of feeling anger? Is there a pattern – are you often angry at the same person in the same situations? If you feel that you are never angry, before you reject the possibility altogether, consider what would be the reaction of another person dealing with your situation. If you think another person might be angry, ask yourself why you feel differently.

So, can we change our feelings about the situations that make us angry?

Jane

Jane is an outgoing, expressive woman who lives with David, a quiet, reserved, intellectual man. The couple get on well, but Jane used to be annoyed by David's apparent secretiveness and expressed her anger by shouting at him. David refused to be drawn into an argument, so Jane would let off steam, then consume any food she could find to calm herself down.

Jane's frustration could only be resolved by learning to appraise her situation in a different way. She was making the mistake of seeing David's secretiveness as a personal criticism. When she began to see it in a different light, as a problem he needed to deal with himself, she was able to remain calmer and consequently eat less. At the same time, as she became less angry with David, he could confide in her more often and the problem began to shrink.

Some experts believe that anger is not caused by the external events that we witness, but by our thoughts about those events. We each see these events in our lives in an individual way, depending on our past experiences and what we have learned from them.

Maxine

Maxine came from a highly critical family. Her father was a university professor and nothing she did was ever good enough for him. She had been overweight for years and, while she managed to achieve many other things in her life, such as becoming a successful solicitor and raising two children while working part-time, she could never keep to a diet. At one point she managed to get almost to her target weight, but just as she was reaching it, a series of family crises caused her eating habits to go haywire. Throughout this time she castigated herself for her 'pathetic' behaviour and ate everything in sight to swallow her anger at herself.

To free herself from this cycle, Maxine had to learn to stop punishing herself for being a failure and abandon her need for everything to be perfect. Once she could allow herself an occasional mistake, the lapses in her diet became less likely to trigger an angry mood swing and the bingeing that followed.

It is not always possible or even appropriate to dispel anger by reframing the situation or paying less attention to what has triggered it. So what do you do when you feel angry, when you need to express your emotions but cannot, because it is not feasible or appropriate to do so? Physical activity, whether it's throwing cushions round the room or going for a brisk swim, can help relieve the physical side-effects of anger and is useful in providing alternative targets. Some people find that immersing themselves in work, or relaxing listening to music, are effective ways of dispelling the tension that comes from angry feelings.

Eating may bring you temporary relief, but only *you* can cure the problem in the long term, by taking control of your actions when you need to release anger, and learning to see the situation differently when you don't.

How to beat cravings and binges

We're all full of the best intentions when we first start dieting. Things seem to be going along swimmingly: the calories are under control, the waistband is definitely a bit looser, and we're feeling pretty good about being so self-disciplined and strong. Then, out of the blue, bang! Your favourite food starts beckoning, in a big way.

Suddenly all your resolve flies out of the window as you make a frantic effort to get your hands on as much of that forbidden food as possible. You feel helpless again, unable to resist the temptation of having a binge. Almost without knowing what's happening, you find yourself standing in the kitchen, madly devouring bar after bar of chocolate, or bowl after bowl of cereal smothered in creamy milk and sugar. The food seems totally irresistible. It's got you in its grip. You tell yourself it's wrong to eat it, but you still can't seem to stop. And you're even aware that you're not really hungry.

All this irrational behaviour, this compulsive overeating, boils down to one thing: you are experiencing and satisfying what is known as a food craving. It's the feeling that you cannot survive without a 'fix'; the substance seems to control you, so that you just have to consume it.

Whether certain foods have power over you because you are addicted to their chemical make-up, or whether you feel compelled to eat them for psychological reasons, is debatable. But its effect on you is the same: you simply lose all rational control and have to eat.

Although we do not know the reasons for these cravings, we do know that they are not instinctive. No baby is born with them. So we must conclude that they are learned behaviour, something we have picked up at some time during our lives. And there lies the hope for everyone who has ever experienced them, because whatever we learn, we can unlearn.

It's vitally important to remember that cravings don't occur in isolation. They don't descend on you out of the blue, although this is how it can feel. Each craving has a trigger, something that prompts you into action. That trigger varies greatly from one person to another. It could be something simple, like the time of day, or something more complex, such as the emotions a certain event always raises. So the first way to start tackling an irrational food craving is to look very carefully for what could be triggering it off.

Next time you feel a craving coming on, stop. Try to identify the feelings going through your mind. Have these thoughts been prompted by a particular emotion? Is it usually this type of event, occurrence or situation that spurs you into a bingeing session?

Then examine the thoughts going through your head. You'll probably notice quite a few imperatives, such as 'I must', and compelling phrases, like 'I should' or 'I ought to'. These kinds of commands make you believe that you have to obey them. And the chances are you will.

Try to switch these phrases around. Say to yourself. 'Perhaps it would be nice to have a sweet/biscuit, etc.' and you'll probably find you no longer feel compelled to have one, because this sort of wording allows you to reply 'Yes, I suppose it would be nice to have a sweet, but actually, I don't really want one at the moment.' By doing this you have allowed yourself a choice.

You should also challenge those imperatives. Ask your-self who told you you should have a sweet. What higher authority is pressing you to have one? Is it really true that there is a compulsion? And if there isn't, why are you obeying a command that has no authority?

Once you start to adopt this questioning approach, you may find that in the minutes it has taken you to think it through, you have lost, or weakened, your craving. Going through this process will also help build up your confidence and prepare you for the next time it happens. And you will have learnt that the craving is not some huge, monstrous thing that's bigger than you. You are bigger than it, and once you realize that, you'll find it easier to question the strength of your craving.

Compulsive behaviour is not only triggered, but can be reinforced. There is always some pay-off involved, some pleasurable experience, no matter how short-lived, that encourages you to do it. And because you feel happier immediately after indulging your compulsion, you continue to do so.

So the key to cracking the compulsion is to look at what surrounds the craving and to break the link between the trigger, the act and the reinforcement. Change one or two things on either side of your behaviour and you're half-way there. It's difficult to generalize about how you should do this, because each individual is unique, with specific triggers and rewards to cope with. But, with careful examination, it can be done.

Another solution is to try to change your external behaviour, so that although deep down you still experience the craving, you don't give in to it. This can be as simple as throwing out your trigger food, refusing to stock it in the house, or making it impossible for you to indulge your compulsion in some other way. Many experts believe that changing the patterns of your physical behaviour (breaking

habits you have acquired) can have a profound
ur thinking process. And they often recommend
l of delving into the deep and often baffling rea-
ou took up the habit in the first place, and why
you continue to have it.

Some extremely effective techniques have been developed to enable you to break the physical habits that are
associated with food cravings. They should also build up
your mental resolve not to give in to a craving. Try the following exercise to see if it helps you.

Exercise

Take a treat that you usually find irresistible. Cut off a piece
of it that's within your daily calorie allowance. Put it on a
plate, then sit down slowly and calmly enjoy your treat as
slowly and seriously as possible. Enjoy it and savour it. At
the same time, examine whether you feel any sense of control at being able to limit yourself to this set amount of
food. Once you have finished eating, quickly move away
and do something completely different. Do this for a few
days, always emphasizing that you're the boss and your
favourite craved food is under your control.

When you are used to this process, take your daily treat
allowance and cut it in two. Throw the other half in the bin.
Tell yourself that you're the one who makes the decisions
about where the food ends up. Then eat the rest of it as
slowly as you can. Congratulate yourself for not putting all
the food in your mouth at once.

Then try something even more testing. Cut your treat in
two, but keep both halves in front of you. When you've finished the first half, get rid of the second half. This should
prove to you that you don't have to eat all of it! Next time,
put your treat on your plate and decide that you don't have
to eat it all. Just see how much you can leave. Try to increase

this amount each day. At first, get rid of the amount left over as soon as you have finished eating. Then try leaving it on the plate to see whether you can still resist it.

Carry out all these strategies in the same place, somewhere you feel calm, secure and in control. Then try them in more difficult situations, when you're on the move, in the car or even in a restaurant. Always make sure that you congratulate yourself for every step forward you have made.

Conquer feelings of failure

If you've tried dieting before, the chances are you're very experienced at goal-setting. Does this sound like you? You have spent a great deal of time thinking about the changes you want to make to your life, and you have even written them all down. Top of your list is to control overeating, to take control of your food intake so that you can lose weight. Second on the list are the 'evil foods' you are going to ban from your life. And you've set yourself a weight-loss target of a stone (6.5 kilos) a month, with the date for reaching your target weight already marked in your diary. While you're at it, you decide to give up tea, coffee and alcohol; and, as you've always meant to give up smoking, you throw away your cigarettes too.

A week later, how are you doing? It's likely that you have broken every single one of your resolutions, so you are back to where you started, except that now you are feeling guilty and miserable about what you see as your failures. You have also reinforced your belief that you can never stick to anything and diets never work for you. Why is it that so many of us seem to set ourselves up for failure in this way?

For many people, the process starts because we are unhappy with ourselves and geuinely want to improve. Our discontentment may stem from a simple acknowledgement that we are out of shape. It could be the result of being bombarded with images of the impossible-to-live-up-to ideals of the perfect body and the superwoman, who always manages her career, family, home and diet superbly and with ease.

Feelings of inadequacy, of not measuring up, could also be the result of a much deeper sense of unhappiness, a feeling so profound that we have difficulty recognizing and coming to terms with it. It is often these emotions that lead us to adopt self-destructive habits in the first place. So it is crucial for us to understand the underlying reasons for our behaviour. Without that basic understanding, we will always find it difficult to change our poor habits.

A bingeing problem, for instance, may not be the cause of our unhappiness (although it undoubtedly makes us unhappy), but a symptom of our unhappiness, masking a root cause we are not able or ready to confront.

If you think this might apply to you, it is really worth trying to examine why you became addicted to chocolate biscuits, cream cakes, chips, or whatever in the first place, and to pinpoint the function that putting food into your mouth serves in your life. Many of us use food to fill emotional gaps in our lives. But what made us feel so empty in the first place? Was it a lack of love, poor self-esteem, or being unable to participate fully in life and surround ourselves with affectionate friends? Is there something fundamentally wrong with our closest relationship that needs attention? Have we suffered a large shock or blow to the ego recently? These could be some of the reasons we turn to food for comfort, but they may not always be obvious to you.

Finding the cause of your behaviour is not an easy task. Talking to a counsellor or a good, sensible friend may help you be more objective about why you react as you do and clarify your hidden motives.

One reason why many of us fail to stick to resolutions therefore, is that we are trying to change the wrong bit of ourselves. We're tinkering with the externals when we should really be going a lot deeper.

Another reason why we fail is that few of us realize what the effects of our new regime will be when we put them into practice. Many successful slimmers say that sticking to 1500 calories a day was the easy part of their diet. The difficult part was coping with the changes this alteration brought to their lives. Once they were no longer 'one of the boys', sinking lagers in the pub, for example, they felt they didn't have much in common with their friends. Giving up their old habits also meant having to look around for other sources of amusement. All this came as a complete shock and took a great deal of adjusting to. Talking to a successful slimmer can help prepare you for the minefield, and she or he can show you ways to cope.

By far the most common cause of failure is setting ourselves goals we cannot possibly achieve. The way to avoid this pitfall is to break down your goals into manageable bits. So, instead of telling yourself that you're going to lose a stone (6.5 kilos) this month, aim to lose a pound (about half a kilo) this week. Just imagine how great you're going to feel if you manage to lose more. That's better than feeling totally defeated by an unattainable goal.

Go on a sensible, healthy diet and reward yourself for every advance you make, no matter how small. Treat yourself like a child. Pat yourself on the back and give yourself a little present or pleasurable experience to celebrate your triumph.

You won't reach your goals if you keep making negative assumptions before you even start. Ask yourself whether negative ideas cross your mind whenever you try to make a decision to diet. Don't think 'I'll never stick to it anyway' or 'I hate salads and couldn't live on rabbit food.'

Thinking like that will undermine your confidence before you even start.

If you feel you need help to achieve your goals, consider joining a support group. Support groups have helped millions curb their bad habits. However, it is absolutely vital that you join the right kind of group. Sometimes people with bad habits get together and do each other no good whatsoever – they just help each other justify their poor behaviour, by blaming everyone and everything else and casting themselves in the role of powerless victims of their habit.

A well-run, positive and sensible support group, such as a Slimming Magazine Club, may provide you with just the kind of help you need during those times when you feel you want to give up and break all your good intentions. But remember that no amount of advice and support will help you lose weight unless you are determined that you want to slim. Resolve that you do, and then stick to your decision.

Free yourself from guilt

At its basic best, guilt is the driving force that makes us take care of our society and pay attention to one another's needs because we feel awful if we don't. It is a deep-rooted internal sense of right and wrong that makes us feel good about ourselves when we act in a responsible or caring way, and bad about ourselves when we do something that we believe to be wrong.

Guilt is not necessarily negative or abnormal in itself, therefore. What really counts is how guilty you feel and what you feel guilty about. There is no doubt that, while some people appear to be born with no sense of social responsibility at all, others are burdened with a very strong guilt streak that makes life needlessly hard for them.

Excessive, misplaced guilt does nothing but harm. It stifles any chance of personal achievement and undermines the development of healthy self-confidence. For a slimmer, it can spell dieting disaster. For example, a slimmer who reacts to any slip-up with wildly exaggerated guilty feelings may have thoughts that go along these lines:

'You are a stupid, hopeless pig. You've let everybody down. You've let yourself down. You don't deserve to be slim. All you deserve is to be a big fat slob, so you may as well go on eating and be a big fat slob!'

Where do these feelings come from? It's very likely that they were formed in early childhood or adolescence. Many children are brought up to equate being acceptable or 'good' with being quiet, unassertive, obedient and, as a consequence, frustrated. Many hear all too clearly the unspoken message that they are not important or valuable as individuals; they are nuisances unless they are being 'good'.

Deep-imprinted guilt can take many disabling forms. Some people grow up with a strong sense that others' needs are far more important than their own. In order to please, they will do anything for anyone, even when it's at the cost of their own well-being and happiness. Some grow up afraid to express their own opinions or to say no when they want to. And some grow up trying to match the impossible ideals that perfectionist and critical parents impressed on them when they were young.

Whatever the cause, overeating is a common escape route from guilty feelings, except that the short-term comfort of eating only leads to more guilty feelings, and the cycle continues. Fortunately, however excessive and disabling, guilt feelings and the black shadow they cast can be conquered, and in a surprisingly short time.

To get you thinking along more positive, guilt-free lines, try the following five strategies.

1 Ask yourself some questions

How do you feel about yourself? If the answer is something like 'Not good. Pretty bad, in fact. I don't see myself as worth much,' ask where this feeling comes from. Bring any old, destructive situations you remember from your childhood out into the light and ask yourself 'How valid were the labels put on me then? And, in any case, why am I still sticking to them now? Am I really so worthless as I've been believing?'

Then consider what would happen if you changed this assessment of yourself. Because it isn't fact. It is a belief – and there's nothing cast in stone to say that it's the fundamental truth about you. The likelihood is that you have been doing yourself less than justice for years. And the exciting thing is that you can change.

2 Let yourself go a little

If you are driven by anxiety to be a high achiever, ask yourself 'Is it sensible to feel this way? Whose standards am I trying to meet? Where did they come from?'

Then, quite deliberately, train yourself to take things a little easier. The world won't fall apart, if, for instance the cupboards aren't spring-cleaned every month, you eat baked beans instead of a Sunday roast once in a while, or your desk at work is not spectacularly neat. You may feel guilty at first for letting previous high standards slip, but if you can practise doing so quite deliberately, you will gradually find you can make life more enjoyable and easier.

3 Practise breaking the rules

If the idea of breaking a diet haunts you, try breaking it *deliberately*. Decide to eat that cream bun or extra bar of chocolate, and say:

'I am doing this quite deliberately, because I am learning that breaking my diet does not make me a bad person. It doesn't make me a failure. I can make a slip like this and go back to my diet without feeling bad. After all, I've only slightly postponed reaching my target weight.'

4 Look out for destructive thoughts

They can catch you out in quite sneaky ways. For instance, if you leave the children with a friend while you and your partner go out for dinner, and the next day you come down with a cold, don't think 'There you are! See what happens when I enjoy myself. This cold serves me right.' If you catch yourself thinking like this even fleetingly, look at your reaction in a cool, reasonable way. You will see that there is no relationship between enjoying yourself and having a cold. You have the same rights as other people and deserve the good things in life just as much as they do.

5 Learn to say no without feeling guilty

If you are too much of a people-pleaser, inclined to keep quiet about your own opinions and to go along with what others want against your own inclinations, you need to practise being more assertive. To begin with, try expressing your thoughts and wishes about relatively unimportant issues. You may feel uncomfortable, but you will be delighted by the way others respond to the more positive you.

How to cope with hunger

When hunger pangs strike, you don't just feel a bit peckish, but as though you haven't eaten for days. They can strike at any time of day – three o'clock in the afternoon, half-past ten in the morning, even in the middle of the night. You know a healthy snack like fresh fruit would be better, but it's all too easy to give in to the lure of a biscuit, a chocolate bar or a bag of crisps. And, come your next meal-time, you'll probably eat as much as usual. So what is the best way of controlling those hunger pangs?

Hunger or appetite?

Hunger can be defined as the body's desire to find and eat food. It is influenced by the body registering that your blood sugar level is low and your stomach is empty. Subconscious influences, such as your mood, also play a part. Satisfying your hunger leads to satiety and is triggered by your senses of taste and smell. It is then influenced by signals from the stomach, intestines and liver, which register that food has been eaten.

The word 'appetite' is used to describe the capacity for eating (as in 'a hearty appetite') or the psychological factors that influence food choice, which are based on habit, social custom, availability of food, environment and personal preference. It's appetite that prompts you to raid the fridge when your body isn't hungry.

Regular is best

Not surprisingly, perhaps, it seems that Nanny knew best: having a regular eating pattern develops the habit of eating only at certain times.

Researchers believe that hunger is influenced by habits and triggers. If you don't have a fixed eating pattern, you may get used to eating when you're not really hungry, and try to resist hunger at other times. This doesn't help the body to feel settled. By establishing a regular eating pattern, the body learns to feel hungry only at certain times and in certain surroundings, such as the dining-room or the kitchen. Stick to a set pattern and see how your feelings of hunger change.

Little and often

If you have three regular meals a day but still suffer from hunger pangs, try eating smaller meals more often. Choose times when you're particularly vulnerable to snacking, such as mid-morning or tea-time. Because there's then less time between meals, you are less likely to snack, and as long as your overall intake is not more than it should be this can be an ideal way to slim.

Change the way you eat

Meal-times used to be family sit-down affairs but nowadays, with our busier lifestyles, meals can often be rushed and unsatisfactory. Yet this aspect of our eating behaviour plays a major role in how full we feel. Snacking and hunger pangs are often just a signal that your mouth hasn't registered that you've eaten, which happens when you've bolted your food without really being aware of it or enjoying it. Set aside time for proper meals and try not to rush them. Eat slowly, chew each mouthful carefully, and it will be more enjoyable and satisfying.

The body takes about 20 minutes before it registers that the stomach is full, so it's easy to finish your meal before your body even knows that it's started. Try starting with less on your plate than usual, but take more time to eat it. Wait a bit and then see how full you really feel.

Eat filling foods

What your meal consists of also determines how full and satisfied you feel. Research has shown that protein has the most satisfying effect on hunger, followed by carbohydrate and then fat. That suggests why it is so easy to overeat on a high-fat diet. Not only does fat contain more calories than any carbohydrate, but it's also less filling and you tend to eat more.

Although protein may have a greater effect on hunger, the ideal diet should still be based on low-fat, high-carbohydrate principles. Foods that are rich in fibre and complex carbohydrates, which are digested more slowly and raise blood-sugar levels more gradually, will stave off hunger pangs for longer.

The Glycaemic Index (GI) is a measure of how quickly a food releases its energy and raises your blood sugar level. The standard food is white bread, with a GI index value of 100. The higher the GI, the higher the food raises your blood sugar level. The more processed and simple a food is, the higher its GI. Honey and puffed rice cereal, for example, have high figures; foods with low GI include wholefoods such as apples, pears, lentils, beans and wholewheat spaghetti. Eating more foods with a low GI will ensure that you have a slow and steady release of energy and help prevent hunger pangs.

Fibre, as both roughage and soluble fibre (such as from oats), is an important factor in GI. It slows down the emptying of your stomach and also swells up slightly, helping you to feel fuller without extra calories.

Keep up the fluids

Drinking plenty of fluids, such as water, is important because it not only gives you a temporary sense of fullness but keeps your body well hydrated, which is vital for general good health. Nutritionists recommend drinking about six to eight glasses of water a day. Drinking regularly will also help prevent symptoms you interpret as hunger pangs that are in fact signs of thirst.

Know your body

If PMS is a problem for you (see below for further information) you may need to increase your calorie intake in the week or so before your period and therefore you may feel hungrier. You may be able to plan for this by keeping an extra-careful eye on the calories in the first two weeks of your cycle, but if hunger pangs really do strike, try to opt for a healthy, filling snack such as a sandwich and a banana instead of a quick-fix chocolate bar or packet of crisps.

Strategies for dealing with PMS

Medical research suggests that around 40 per cent of all women of child-bearing age may seriously suffer from premenstrual syndrome (PMS), with its varied physical and emotional symptoms that can cause real distress to a woman and those closest to her. But there is a lot of evidence that many more women are adversely affected to a lesser extent for a few days before a period. These milder symptoms can range from feeling more weepy, irritable or tired than usual to comfort-eating or having cravings for chocolate or other high-sugar foods, all of which can make sticking to a diet that much harder.

Of course, it comes as no surprise that comfort-eating and feeling tense go hand in hand, but in the case of PMS there seems to be a well-founded link between the amount of food we eat and the menstrual cycle itself. Research shows that women do tend to eat more, and particularly more sweet foods, in the second half of their cycle than in the first half.

If you recognize this pattern in yourself, it's worth preparing for it by being extra strict with your diet in the two weeks or so after a period in order to allow yourself to indulge more in the two weeks before.

The complex links between overeating and other PMS symptoms are based on hormonal changes that take place in the body throughout the menstrual cycle. There is therefore a body-chemistry cause for severe PMS, although symptoms vary enormously. Psychological symptoms include mood swings, irritability, lethargy, nervous tension, anxiety and depression. Physical ones include food cravings, headaches and migraines, feeling bloated, clumsiness and temporary weight gain due to water retention.

You'll notice that these symptoms mostly echo the ailments that can affect us at any time for any reason. So if you think that you and your dieting are seriously affected by PMS, it's important to get a proper diagnosis. It may be that you do not have PMS at all, but some other problem that can be treated successfully.

To help with any diagnosis of PMS, try keeping a day-by-day symptom diary for at least three months, noting such troublesome things as lack of energy, food cravings, mood swings, and so on. If you find that, on the whole, you are normally cheerful and capable but suffer some disagreeable mental or physical problems in the week or two before a period, try these self-help tips:

● Check up on your basic eating

If you are intending to lose any surplus weight on a healthy diet, you will automatically be doing a lot to lessen any PMS problems. There's considerable evidence to show that PMS symptoms are much reduced if sufferers (whether slimming or not) switch to healthier eating habits, ensuring a balanced supply of all the vitamins and minerals the body needs to function properly.

You can probably recite the healthy-eating guidelines in your sleep, but here they are again: base your diet on wholegrain bread, pasta, cereals, fruit, vegetables, fish, lean meat and modest amounts of low-fat dairy products.

● Look at your lifestyle

Here too you probably already know the important things to do for a healthier lifestyle: give up smoking, keep alcohol levels to no more than 14 units a week, and become more physically active in every way you can think of. Walking, dancing, running, swimming, keep-fit classes, etc. will pay really big rewards in terms of fitness, vitality and lightened mood throughout the month. Watch your stress levels too (see below for further information on this).

● Expect a monthly shock from the scales

One of the more common symptoms of PMS is a feeling of being uncomfortably bloated and heavy; the scales may even show a sudden increase in weight of between 2 pounds and 4 pounds (1 and 2 kilos). This does not mean that a faithfully followed diet is not working, so don't panic or despair. The gain is a strictly temporary one, due to fluid retention prompted by hormonal changes, and should disappear once your period has started. In the mean time, many women find it helps to cut out or at least cut down on salt.

● Forgive your PMS 'sins'

If you are keeping to a healthy slimming diet for the rest of the month, a few indulgences at PMS time may slightly delay Target Day but won't prevent you succeeding in the end. In fact, depriving yourself of chocolate or biscuits when you most crave them could be counter-productive.

Instead of munching through a huge, full-milk chocolate bar, though, try snacks such as a reduced-calorie hot chocolate drink and a low-fat chocolate bar, which many chocaholics find enough to satisfy a craving.

● Get disruptive symptoms taken seriously

Most doctors take PMS seriously, but if your GP isn't particularly helpful ask to be referred for specialist help. Research shows that some PMS sufferers (but not all) benefit from taking evening primrose oil or other supplements, but before self-medicating it is worth getting proper professional advice.

● Advance planning pays

With time you can develop coping strategies for PMS, for example planning to take extra exercise if you know you are likely to be irritable, pampering yourself if you feel tired and down, or trying to avoid scheduling major work projects if you know you may not be feeling super-efficient.

Like any other problem, PMS loses a lot of its power to plague you when given a long, cool look.

Boost your self-esteem

Do you tend to be very critical and judgemental of yourself and others? Are you always rushing around trying to please everyone? Do you sometimes feel as though the world is against you? If any of these sounds familiar, chances are you have low self-esteem, and this is one of the factors that may contribute to a weight problem.

To realize how damaging low self-esteem can be, it's important to understand the difference between self-esteem and confidence. You can put on a show of confidence – many of us do – but it is only superficial. This is the difference between confidence and self-esteem: confidence can be feigned, but you can't pretend to feel good about yourself.

For example, if your confidence is dented – perhaps by a tactless comment, an upset in the family, or a reprimand at work – a high level of self-esteem acts like a buffer, keeping your confidence high and helping you to cope. If your self-esteem is basically low, there's nothing to boost your confidence when you're faced with one of life's knocks.

Trying to keep your confidence high without the support of self-esteem can be very demanding, so we find artificial props to fill the gap between our low self-esteem and the veneer of confidence we want to present to the world. Some people drink too much, others take drugs, or keep themselves frantically busy; others again resort to food. But these addictions only make matters worse. Overeating just confirms your poor opinion of yourself, so your self-esteem falls even lower.

The answer is to try to increase your self-esteem so that you are not dependent on food to fill the gaps – but how? If you have low self-esteem, you usually tend to bottle up your negative emotions instead of facing up to them. You may turn to food for comfort when you feel distressed or overtired, but want to put on a happy face to the world. When you do this you're using food to bolster your confidence and help you cope with everyday life.

Recognizing your feelings – negative and positive – is an important step towards raising your self-esteem. Rather than forcibly silencing your emotions with food, allow yourself to deal with them, whether it means sitting down for a good cry right away or containing your anger until a more suitable time, then releasing it.

This may be hard if showing strong feelings of any kind was discouraged or even frowned upon in your family, but you can learn a lot from more tempestuous types who throw cushions around or cry at sentimental films. Once you begin to let your emotions show, it's easier to feel strong on the inside, and to resist the temptation to overeat.

It's also important to remember you have a choice. Try to be aware of those times when you are thinking negative thoughts about yourself or others. Be honest with yourself about what's going on and then tell yourself that you can either sit there and moan, blaming others or feeling sorry for yourself (in which case you may well reinforce your feelings of guilt, anxiety or resentment with food) – or you can do something about it.

It may take courage to make changes – whether this involves going on a diet or changing jobs – but, if it means enough to you, you can do it.

By simply acknowledging that you have a choice, you are going a long way towards releasing the springs of self-esteem that you have been holding down, allowing them to boost your confidence. When your confidence is propped up naturally with self-esteem, there's no longer a gap to be filled artificially with food – and you'll feel a lot better about yourself and the people around you.

Ten steps to better self-esteem

1 Stop putting yourself down. None of us is perfect. Your friends and family all have their own weaknesses, but you can still love them, so why is it so hard to love yourself? Try to accept your faults and be more tolerant towards yourself.

2 Distract your attention away from a poor body image by concentrating on yourself as a person. Try this exercise: sit in front of a mirror in a candle-lit room and imagine that you are meeting the person in the mirror for the first time. Hold a conversation and see what comes back to you. Find out all about that person. Meet her for the first time without thinking about her size. She's extremely likeable, isn't she?

3 Wake up to all the good things around you. If you have low self-esteem it's easy to get so entrenched with your negative feelings that you shut everything else out, like compliments from your partner and friends. Climb out of the victim hole and start appreciating what's going on around you.

4 Take up some form of exercise. There's a connection between your energy levels and emotional levels: if you feel good about your body, you'll feel better in yourself.

5 Get creative, whether it's sewing, writing, dancing, drawing, singing or cooking. Doing something creative offers a challenge and sense of achievement and has a very real effect on how you feel about yourself.

6 Give your body the love and attention it deserves. Treat yourself to a manicure or massage, buy some sexy underwear or sensual perfume. Indulge yourself!

7 Try new horizons. Break your routine. Go to shops that you've never been in before, try new foods, speak to new people. There's a new exciting world out there, just waiting to be discovered.

8 Cultivate your friendships. Write someone a letter; ring up someone you've not spoken to for ages. It's good to talk!

9 Make space for yourself. Stop being someone's mother, wife, sister or secretary for a few minutes and get back in touch with your true identity. Remind yourself who you are and what you need.

10 Take time out to relax. Learn a technique to help you calm down and get rid of stress.

How to stop smoking and slim

Few people can be unaware of how dangerous smoking is to health, but many smokers who also want to slim are afraid to give up because they worry that stopping smoking will cause them to put on weight. In surveys, weight gain is an often quoted reason for ex-smokers taking up the habit again, and women in particular tend to believe that smoking actually keeps them slim.

An extensive US study found that women did in fact gain about 7 pounds (3 kilos) and men about 5 pounds (2 kilos) on average when they quit smoking. More worryingly, one in eight women and one in ten men put on over 2 stone (12.5 kilos).

However, put in the context of your overall health, it looks like a very false economy to continue smoking in the belief that it will prevent weight gain. First, there is no medical evidence that this is the case. In fact, many smokers also have a weight problem. But there's a great deal of evidence to prove that smoking kills. Every hour thirteen people in the UK die from a smoking-related disease, the big killers being lung cancer, heart disease and stroke. There is also the more general fact that smokers are more lethargic, unfit and prone to illness than those who don't smoke. The health benefits of not smoking far outweigh the risks of putting on weight, but many of us ignore those benefits if there is even a slight chance we might put on weight.

Why do we put on weight when we stop smoking? One much-quoted theory is that metabolic rate increases when you smoke and slows down again when you quit, and it's your metabolic rate that governs how quickly your body burns energy, otherwise known as calories. Research has found that this isn't true for all and the increase is small – equivalent to about 100 calories a day – but this could be enough to cause slow, gradual weight gain for some.

A more significant factor is much more simple: we eat more. Some people, when deprived of a cigarette, look around for another pleasure or crutch, and it's usually food or drink. Secondly, the empty feelings of nicotine withdrawal are similar to hunger pangs, and smokers who are quitting tend to start shovelling food down to get rid of these feelings. The body will have recovered from withdrawal symptoms within five to seven days, but by that time you may be used to overeating, and will carry on doing so. A weight problem can result.

The problem is made worse by the fact that food often tastes better once you stop smoking, as your senses of taste and smell return. And if the food that suddenly tastes even more wonderful is chocolate, it's not surprising that weight gain may result.

Weight gain is not inevitable if you make a firm decision to give up smoking, accept that you may be tempted to turn to food and draw up a battle plan to stop yourself giving in to it. Try these five strategies to help:

1 Plan for feeling hungrier

Create daily menus that are big on filling foods, such as jacket potatoes, pasta, stews and soups. Have healthy snacks ready to eat (fruit, raw vegetable sticks, crispbreads or rice cakes, low-fat or diet yogurt, sugar-free chewing gum, even the occasional packet of low-fat crisps).

2 Take control of your thoughts

Don't think of giving up smoking in terms of sacrifice; concentrate on all the positive benefits you will enjoy from being a non-smoker. Tell yourself that any hungry withdrawal feelings are not real hunger but the body ridding itself of poison. Once the withdrawal symptoms are over, you will never have to experience them again.

If there are situations – at the pub, dining out or watching television, for instance – that you find difficult, devise strategies to combat them. For example, if you find the post-meal craving for a cigarette unbearable, don't stay at the table. Try getting up as soon as you've finished eating, to clear the table and wash up.

3 Get some exercise

It can help to overcome cravings by channelling your thoughts and energy in another direction. It makes you feel good in yourself, and helps you burn off any extra calories you may be taking in. Swimming, aerobics, cycling or jogging are all excellent but if you feel you can't manage anything so strenuous, try getting exercise in small ways, such as walking instead of taking the car on short journeys, gardening, using the stairs instead of lifts or escalators, or walking the dog twice a day instead of once.

4 Capitalize on the plus side of giving up

If food tastes better, try out some new low-fat or low-calorie recipes. Use the money you save on cigarettes for a special (non-food!) treat, such as clothes, a book, perfume or a CD. Make a list of all the good things that will come out of giving up smoking, from fresher breath and more energy to lowering your risk of stroke and cancer, and place it somewhere prominent as a reminder of all the reasons you decided to give up.

5 Get help

If giving up smoking and maintaining your weight seem just too tough on your own, try joining a support group such as a Slimming Magazine Club where you'll find advice and motivation on the diet side of your campaign. For advice and support while giving up smoking, phone Quitline on 0800 002200.

How to beat stress

We all need quite a lot of the right sort of stress in our lives, the kind that keeps us on our toes, and produces the excitement and interest that enable us to meet challenges and welcome opportunities for our own personal growth.

If we were never faced with any situations which demanded decisions and action – for example, if we found ourselves forcibly confined to one room with no need to lift a finger but without entertainment or stimulation – it wouldn't be long before we were suffering from very severe stress of the wrong sort.

When stress is used to describe a state of feeling pressured and emotionally fragmented, it can be a very threatening word, one that can tyrannize and push us around. Thinking of stress in this way can mean that we allow ourselves to be brainwashed into thinking that certain situations and events must make us 'stress victims'. And it's disconcerting if other situations that we genuinely do find stressful don't seem to be highly rated in so-called stress comparison charts.

The view that stress and strain are automatically built into certain situations has been reinforced in many people's minds by a frequently quoted table which rates such events as divorce, having babies, switching jobs, moving house and driving in traffic jams according to how much stress each is supposed to induce.

Yet getting married, moving house and switching jobs (all of which are highly rated for stress on these tables) can charge many people with surges of excitement and energy rather than anxiety and anguish. The arrival of babies and bringing up children are not inevitably stressful. Many parents find that their children's baby years are among the happiest and the most rewarding. It's brainwashed thinking that makes us say things like: 'That poor woman works terribly long hours and must be under awful pressure' or 'I don't know why that girl can't stick to a diet. She has a wonderful job, and nobody to cater for except herself.'

But people who work long hours may well do so because they love their work, or because the end goal they have in mind makes the pressures exciting and productive. An unsuccessful slimmer may have real dieting difficulties based on a number of stressful factors which aren't apparent to an outsider. She may have problems with her partner, her manager or her parents. She may be trying to slim in order to please somebody else, or because friends have been telling her she ought to, and she's failing because it isn't something she wants to do for herself.

Stress is very personal, and stress factors simply aren't the same for everyone. The people, situations and encounters that give you stress may be quite different from those that affect your best friend. This is why it's vital not to be afraid of the word, and never to feel that, because other people can and do cope in your situation, you should be able to (and vice versa).

The really important thing is to try to recognize when you yourself are under too much stress. Check out the list of early-warning stress symptoms below. If you have three or more and can't see your way out of them, there is a strong chance that you are under too much of the wrong kind of stress.

- Becoming easily tired
- Often feeling vaguely off-colour
- Having a lot of minor aches and pains
- Not sleeping as normal
- Comfort-eating much more than usual
- Going off the idea of food
- Finding the present unsatisfying and the future frightening
- Diverting energy from important things to fuss over lots of little things
- Dithering; finding even simple decisions overwhelming
- Feeling bored about today, this evening and tomorrow
- Being unusually short-tempered and irritable
- Drinking and/or smoking more than usual
- Finding it harder and harder to take time off

Stress-busting techniques

• Pay attention to your health

It is much easier to deal with stressful situations when we are feeling physically fit. So resist the temptation to take the easy way out by drinking or smoking too much, overeating or neglecting exercise and relaxation. It's particularly important to eat healthily, make time for at least a brisk walk in the fresh air every day, and get enough sleep.

● Take action towards obvious improvements

Think about what you would *really* like to change in your life, and focus on the changes that you want for yourself, not for others or because you feel you 'ought to'. Remember that a reluctant dieter who is slimming under protest is actually causing herself stress. Provided you are making the effort because you actively want to be slimmer and healthier, steady progress towards your target will diminish stress as you start feeling in far better control of yourself.

● Accept what you can't change

There are always going to be temporarily stressful situations that you can't alter. Decide now that you will make a conscious effort not to add to your problems by getting 'in a state'. Decide to reserve your energy for situations you *can* save. And remember that it often isn't the situation itself that is stressful: it is your attitude to it.

● Do one thing at a time

When life seems to be asking too much of you in any area, what you have to do is make a list of all the things you do in order of priority, and then *put yourself first*. Ask: 'To me, what are the most important things on my agenda? And what are the least important?' If you decide to stay clear-headed and guilt-free about all this, you should find that you can knock some items off your list immediately and delegate or share others.

● Recognize the stressful power of resentment

People who live with a permanent state of resentment boiling away inside can make themselves ill. Bottled-up strong emotions are corrosive. So it's vital to confront situations or behaviour that make you resentful.

• Your self-respect is more important than somebody else's displeasure

People who are too compliant for their own good may well have got the idea in childhood that standing up for themselves meant being branded as unlovable. But if you want to avoid all the stress that comes from frustrated wishes and bottled-up feelings, you must learn to be assertive. Say to yourself: 'This is my own individual independence and self-respect that is at stake,' and you will find it easier to come straight out with what you want to say. Very often you will find that the outcome is much better than you had fearfully imagined – and you will feel better about yourself as a result.

• Allow yourself to be human

When you make a mistake, as we all do occasionally, see it as a learning opportunity, not a reason for criticizing yourself for not being perfect. Human beings *aren't* perfect. So instead of giving yourself a hard time for breaking your diet, losing your temper or failing an interview, say: 'I made a mess of it. Too bad. I'll learn from that and next time I'll cope much better.' Training yourself to look at things in this positive way will reduce your stress load a lot.

• Cherish your lines of communication

Poor communication, mistaken assumptions and lack of mutual understanding can lead to very stressful situations and relationships at work, in families and among friends. Take time to learn and respect other people's tastes and opinions, and try to make sure other people know yours.

● Switch off every day in your own way

Whether or not you feel under stress at the moment, the golden rule is to find some way of relaxing that you enjoy, and take at least fifteen minutes every single day to enjoy it. Some people like to learn techniques such as meditation or yoga, others find more vigorous exercise helpful, while others again prefer quieter pursuits like listening to music, reading a novel, or having a luxurious bath. Spending time with a special person who makes you laugh and relaxes you is great, and even watching television is OK as long as you find it genuinely relaxing and not mildly boring or irritating. Whatever works for you, make time for it every day, even when you feel you haven't time – *especially* when you feel you haven't time.

3

The safe and successful way to slim

This section of *Dare to Bare* aims to give you the tools or building blocks you need to find your own, successful way to lose weight and keep it off.

It begins with '*How to lose weight, eat well and stay healthy*', which includes a foolproof way to ensure your diet is balanced and contains the vitamins, minerals and nutrients you need. We then look in more detail at several components of the average diet that are particularly relevant to slimming healthily, to ask '*Are you getting enough – or too much?*'

To slim successfully, it's essential to find a way of controlling your energy intake that feels comfortable for you. '*Two ways to slim*' explains the two main ways to achieve this: counting fat, and counting calories, and how to make each work for you.

The last part of this section focuses you clearly on what target weight you should be aiming for, and how to work out the level of energy intake that will set you safely and steadily on the road to success.

How to lose weight, eat well and stay healthy

Before planning a diet that will help you lose weight its important to be aware of the overall principles that can ensure you are eating a balanced diet with enough vitamins, minerals and other nutrients.

Slimming's formula for planning a diet agrees very much with *The Balance of Good Health*, the latest Government National Food Guide. This was developed by the Department of Health, the Health Education Authority and the Ministry of Agriculture, Fisheries and Food.

The Balance of Good Health divides foods into five groups: Fruit and Vegetables; Bread, Cereals and Potatoes; Milk and Dairy Foods; Meat, Fish, and Alternatives; and Foods containing fat/sugar. Each day, you should aim to have certain number of servings from each of the groups. *Slimming* recommends the following:

- **Five** servings of different fruit and vegetables.
- **Four** servings of bread, pasta, cereals, potatoes, or rice. Aim to have one serving at each meal.
- **Three** servings of milk and dairy products. Choose low-fat varieties where possible.
- **Two** servings of meat, fish, eggs, beans, nuts or meat alternatives. Choose lean or low-fat varieties where possible.
- **Extras and Treats:** sweets, alcohol, biscuits, cake, chocolate etc are optional extras; limit your intake and have no more than **ONE** small serving per day.

These guidelines apply to teenagers, adults, children over five, vegetarians, and those who are overweight.

Thinking of food in groups in this way gives you the building blocks for devising the diet that will suit you best. Whichever kind of diet you choose, you can plan your daily menus so that the bulk of your food intake comes from the two largest groups; that you include several servings of milk, dairy products and meat, fish and alternatives each day, and that you limit your intake from the extras group.

The great thing about this approach is that no food need be forbidden; you can include all your favourites as long as you plan for them within your overall diet.

However, it's important to look a bit more closely at some of the constituents of these food groups to check that you are getting enough (or not having too much!) in certain areas of your diet.

Successful slimming tip: don't forget to drink!

To stay fit and healthy and to help with your dieting campaign, it's vital to have plenty to drink. Liquids keep the body well-hydrated, which is important for good health, and drinking plenty of low-calorie fluids will help fill you up and reduce hunger pangs. Nutritionists recommend drinking between six and eight glasses of water every single day. Alternatively, drink tea and coffee (with milk from your dairy allowance and sweetener), diet soft drinks, Marmite or Bovril.

Are you getting enough vitamins and minerals?

Antioxidants

Antioxidants include vitamins A (beta carotene), C and E, known as the 'ACE' vitamins. There is also evidence that some minerals, such as selenium, zinc and copper, are antioxidants.

In the body, antioxidants affect oxidation, the same process that causes cars to rust. It happens in our bodies all the time, and produces potentially harmful agents called free radicals. Free radicals are created naturally as a by-product of reactions in our body, but if we are exposed to environmental pollutants, such as car fumes or cigarette smoke, we produce more. There is strong evidence to suggest that antioxidants protect against too many free radicals being produced in the body. They are believed to have a neutralizing effect, mopping up the free radicals.

If the production of free radicals in our bodies increases (as a result of smoking, for example), a chain reaction starts which generates more and more free radicals. These molecules can damage cells and the genetic material they contain. This process is thought to be at least partly to blame for chronic diseases such as cancer. Free radicals are believed to increase the likelihood of cholesterol being deposited in the arteries, which can lead to heart disease.

Fruit and vegetables are two of the best sources of antioxidant vitamins.

- Good sources of beta carotene (which the body converts into vitamin A) include green leafy vegetables, broccoli and yellow-orange vegetables and fruit.
- Good sources of vitamin A include liver, cod liver oil, cheese and eggs.
- Vitamin C is found in citrus fruit (such as oranges) and several other fruit and vegetables.
- Good sources of vitamin E are nuts, vegetable oils and wholemeal bread.

Government guidelines recommend that we all eat five portions of fruit and vegetables every day. Potatoes don't count towards these five portions, although pulses such as peas, beans (including baked beans) and lentils, do.

In general, one portion represents a piece of fruit, a small glass of fruit juice, a large salad or a 75 g (3 oz) serving of vegetables. The vegetables in a casserole, for example, would count as one portion.

The Reference Nutrient Intake (RNI) of some of the antioxidant mutrients for adult men and women's daily needs is:

- Vitamin A: 600 ug (0.6 mg). To make one unit of vitamin A, the body needs six units of beta carotene. Very high doses of vitamin A, especially from animal sources such as liver, should be avoided by pregnant women, as should supplements containing Vitamin A unless prescribed by a doctor.
- Vitamin C: 40 mg. An orange has 80 mg of vitamin C. If you smoke you should have extra vitamin C for example, an extra orange or glass of orange juice per day.
- Vitamin E : more than 4 mg. A 100 gram (3½ ounce) portion of boiled spinach contains 1.7 mg of vitamin E. There are no proven toxic effects of high intakes of vitamin C and E, but massive consumption of foods high in beta carotene (such as carrots) may turn the skin yellow!

If you eat a varied healthy diet, you can get all the antioxidants you need from food, and therefore should not need special supplements except under medical advice.

Calcium

Calcium is a mineral which is an essential component of our bone structure; it accounts for about 2 per cent of our body weight. Children need calcium for the growth of their bones and teeth, and adults need it to keep bones and teeth healthy. Although we stop growing, we never outgrow our need for calcium.

Your requirement for calcium varies according to your age and sex; government recommendations are 700 mg per day or more for all adults. As a guide, 275 ml (half a pint) of skimmed milk has 340 mg of calcium (the same amount of whole milk has 325 mg). A 150 gram (5½ ounce) pot of low-fat natural yogurt contains 285 mg, and 25 grams (1 ounce) of reduced-fat Cheddar cheese has 235 mg calcium. A 115 gram (4 ounce) portion of boiled spinach has 185 mg of calcium and a 150 gram (5½ ounce) can of baked beans has 80 mg. Sardines, spring greens, oranges, broccoli and bread are also quite good sources.

If you don't eat enough calcium-rich foods regularly, you may be at risk of developing osteoporosis (brittle bone disease) in later life. As a normal part of the ageing process, calcium is lost from the bone faster than its replaced. The bones gradually lose their strength and become more brittle. If we lose too much calcium the result is osteoporosis, a condition in which the bones become so weak that they break. We reach our peak bone mass at around the age of 30. After this, more calcium is lost from our bones than is absorbed. It is essential that we eat plenty of calcium-rich foods in our teens and twenties to ensure that, as we get older, we have enough calcium in the bank to keep our bones strong despite the inevitable loss of bone mass.

Women are more vulnerable than men to osteoporosis because of the hormonal changes that occur around the menopause. Levels of oestrogen, one of the hormones that help bone to retain its strength, fall around this time and the rate of loss of calcium and bone mass increases substantially. So the greater our bone mass to start off with, the better. Hormone replacement therapy (HRT) in middle-aged women can delay this onset of loss of bone mass.

To prevent osteoporosis, the best thing you can do is start early, by eating calcium-rich foods regularly to ensure your bones are at their strongest at the age of 30. But, whatever age you are, it's important to continue to eat calcium-rich foods.

Other osteoporosis-beating tips include:

- Get plenty of exercise as this strengthens bones and helps prevent calcium loss.
- Avoid drinking large amounts of alcohol. It reduces calcium absorption.
- Quit smoking. Smoking can affect your hormones and so have the same effect as menopause on your bones.
- Get plenty of fresh air. We cannot absorb calcium without the help of vitamin D, the vitamin our skin manufactures naturally when it is exposed to sunlight.

The best sources of calcium are milk, cheese and yogurt reduced-fat varieties contain similar amounts to full-fat versions. Calcium from these foods is easily absorbed and supplies over half our daily calcium intake. Foods such as spinach and nuts are high in calcium, but in a form that is not as easily absorbed.

Iron

Iron is a mineral we assume we've got covered, especially those of us who eat meat, as it's a rich source of iron. But some sections of the population may be, at best, borderline deficient in iron, with many people not even taking in enough iron necessary to keep healthy and ward off the debilitating symptoms of anaemia.

Iron deficiency particularly affects teenage girls and women, because they may suffer high iron losses every month with their period. It may even be difficult for women who have very heavy periods to replace the lost iron through diet alone, especially if they are vegetarian. Sometimes supplements are needed.

Vegetarians may be more likely to be iron-deficient because vegetarian sources of iron, like green leafy vegetables, bread, fortified cereals and beans, provide so-called non-haem iron, which the body cannot use as easily as haem iron, which is found in red meat and offal. One of the vital ingredients in this process is vitamin C, which helps the body to use non-haem iron, so vegetarians need to get a good supply of non-meat sources of iron and vitamin C, combining them in the same meal: for example, a glass of orange juice with a bowl of breakfast cereal, or fruit after a sandwich.

Why is iron deficiency such a cause for concern? Iron is responsible for carrying oxygen around the body, as haemoglobin in blood and myoglobin in muscles. If our need for iron outstrips supply, and stores are used up, oxygen is no longer being carried efficiently around the body and symptoms of iron-deficiency anaemia develop: fatigue, muscle weakness, pale skin, breathlessness, light-headedness and poor concentration. Other signs can include frequent mouth ulcers, curving brittle fingernails, reduced hair growth, stomach problems like indigestion, and tingling in fingers and toes. In addition, because lack of iron stops the immune system working effectively, you're more likely to suffer from colds and infections.

For children, the situation is more critical because iron is vital for physical growth and mental development, particularly balance, language and learning skills. Iron deficiency is associated with lower results in intelligence tests and a poorer overall school performance. Several studies have found that the effect of iron deficiency on development is irreversible, even after a child's iron status is back up to par.

For all these reasons, it's vital that all the family get a good iron intake through their diet. If you get a good dietary supply you shouldn't need to take supplements, but if you are concerned, it's a good idea to see your GP. A simple blood test to check your haemoglobin levels will tell you whether you have an iron deficiency or not, and then you can be prescribed supplements if necessary.

The good news is that there's no reason why you should run low on iron when you're slimming, as long as you plan your diet to include iron-rich foods. To be sure you're getting enough, choose red meat and offal, particularly liver and kidney; green, leafy vegetables; beans and pulses; wholemeal bread, nuts, and fortified breakfast cereals.

Vitamin C, which helps in iron absorption, is found in citrus fruit and juices, particularly blackcurrants and berry fruits such as strawberries; vegetables like Brussels sprouts, broccoli and cauliflower, tomatoes, peppers and new potatoes.

Fat

Fat has the reputation of being the slimmer's worst enemy – these days almost everyone is aware of the need to reduce the amount of fat we eat.

In fact, you do need *some* fat in your diet; fat is essential to enable your body to function healthily and provides the important fat-soluble vitamins (A,D,E, and K) and also provides essential fatty acids which can't be made in the body and have to be supplied in the diet. But, apart from helping you to slim, there is another good reason to reduce your fat intake: a high fat intake in your diet (particularly saturated fat) may be linked to heart disease and some cancers.

Reducing the total amount of fat you eat can help lower a high blood cholesterol level, which is one of the risk factors for heart disease. In addition to reducing your total fat intake, you should also consider the type of fat you eat.

Fats can be divided into three groups, according to their chemical make-up: saturates (so-called 'bad fats'), polyunsaturates and monounsaturates (so-called 'good fats'). You should aim to eat moderate amounts of foods that are high in polyunsaturates and monounsaturates (for example, oily fish, such as mackerel, sardine and herring; and olive, corn and safflower oils). At the same time, cut down foods high in saturates (including fatty meats and meat products and full-fat dairy foods, such as butter, whole milk and cream). Cakes, biscuits, chocolate, puddings, pastry, fried foods, crisps etc can also be high is saturates.

Fats are higher in calories than any other type of food – good news for slimmers, because it means that if you cut down on fat, you're sure to lose weight. The fats in food actually contain about twice the calories of carbohydrates or proteins. No wonder foods high in fat are high in calories too!

So reducing the amount of fat in your diet and increasing the amount of carbohydrate is an important key to losing weight. And you needn't keep such a detailed eye on the calories, either.

The logic behind this is that excess calories from fats are more likely to be stored in the body as fat than excess calories from carbohydrates. If you overeat on high-carbohydrate foods (potatoes, cereals, pasta, rice and bread) the surplus calories are stored as glycogen, which remains in the liver and muscle until needed as a source of energy. Only when the stores are full is excess carbohydrate converted to fat.

A high-carbohydrate, low-fat diet makes it difficult to eat too much because it is very bulky and satisfying. Fats, on the other hand, increase the palatability of food so that it tastes better, but they're less satisfying, which means its far easier to overeat. Imagine how many pieces of bread and butter you could eat when you're hungry. Would you eat as many without the butter? Probably not!

It isn't always obvious just which foods are high in fat. When we talk about fats, we don't only mean the tub of margarine or bottle of oil you keep in the fridge. There are lots of foods that contain hidden fats, some naturally-occurring such as in peanuts and avocados, and some added during processing or manufacturing, for instance to ready made meals, sauces, pastries and chocolate.

Five easy low fat switches

1 Change to low-fat dairy products, such as skimmed milk, reduced-fat cheese, low-fat or diet yogurts and fromage frais; and switch from butter or margarine to low-fat spread (better still, don't use any spread!).
2 Always buy lean meat or reduced-fat meat products, such as lean minced beef and low-fat sausages.
3 Never fry foods – always grill, poach, steam, boil or bake. Dry-fry minced meat.
4 Always buy tinned fish in brine or tomato sauce, not oil.
5 Skim the fat off stews and casseroles before you serve them.

Fibre

Dietary fibre is a mixture of the carbohydrates found in fruits, vegetables and other plant products, such as wheat. Dietary fibre cannot be completely digested and so passes straight through the body, making up much of the content of the stools. As a result, it also helps to keep your bowel movements regular.

There are two types of fibre: insoluble and soluble. Insoluble fibre is found mainly in pasta, some breakfast cereals, bran and some vegetables. Soluble fibre is present in virtually all fruits and vegetables, but pulses (peas, beans and lentils) and oats are the main sources.

Experts say adults should eat around 18 grams (about half an ounce) of fibre every day for good health. This could come from: 25 grams (1 ounce) of bran flakes; two medium slices of wholemeal bread; a 150 gram (5½ ounce) can of baked beans; an apple, or an orange. (The calorie count of all this food, incidentally, is only 465 calories).

Fibre is good for us because insoluble fibre helps to keep bowel movements regular, preventing constipation. Research has shown that people with a high fibre intake have a lower risk of bowel cancer. Soluble fibre is thought to help lower cholesterol levels, thereby reducing the risk of heart disease. Foods rich in fibre, such as fruit and vegetables, tend to be low in calories, which is good news for slimmers. But they also offer other benefits. High-fibre foods are often bulky and make you feel full up more quickly than other foods. Fibre also slows down the rate at which sugar is absorbed, and high-fibre foods tend to stay in your stomach longer, both of which effects mean that you will feel fuller for longer.

The best way to eat more fibre is to increase the amount of fibre in your diet gradually. If you eat too much too quickly, you may experience discomfort. It is important to drink plenty of water when you increase your fibre intake. Fibre is like a sponge – it soaks up a lot of fluid, and then expands in your stomach, giving you a full-up feeling. Eating a lot of fibre without drinking enough may cause constipation.

Here are some easy ways to get more fibre:

- Start the day with a wholewheat cereal, or one containing bran or oats.
- Swap white bread for wholemeal.
- Eat vegetables with their skins on.
- Replace some of the meat in your diet with beans or lentils (in casseroles, for example).
- Eat plenty of fruit.

Salt

Most of us add salt to some foods, whether its during cooking or at the table. But there is far more hidden salt in many of the foods we buy, which can make it difficult to control your intake.

Salt, or sodium chloride, is our most common source of sodium, which is vitally important to the body as it helps maintain fluid volumes and, therefore, blood pressure. Sodium is also needed for the transmission of nerve and muscle impulses, as well as for the uptake of certain nutrients in the small intestine.

A gram of salt contains 0.4 grams of sodium, and the requirement we need for health is 1.6 grams sodium a day, which is equivalent to around 4 grams of salt (less than a teaspoonful). However, in the UK we consume more salt than we need. Men take in about 10 grams of salt a day on average, and women about 7.5 grams a day. This means an average sodium intake of much more than we need.

Scientific evidence shows that sodium (and therefore salt) intake can affect blood pressure, and experts believe that high intakes of sodium (more than 3.2 grams a day) may lead to raised blood pressure in susceptible people. High blood pressure can increase your risk of strokes or heart disease. Research also shows that reducing your salt intake can help reduce raised blood pressure levels, especially in conjunction with other diet and lifestyle changes such as keeping a healthy body weight, getting plenty of exercise and cutting down on alcohol.

The sodium in our diet comes from three main sources: 15 to 20 per cent comes from salt added during cooking and at table, and 15 per cent comes from sodium naturally present in some foods, but 60 to 70 per cent comes from salt added to foods during manufacture or processing, as a preservative or to improve flavour or texture.

As a guide, a 50 g (2 oz) portion of salted peanuts has 0.2 g of sodium, 25 g (1 oz) Cheddar cheese has 0.17 g of sodium, 15 ml (1 tbsp) sweet pickle has 0.68 g of sodium and one rasher of grilled bacon has 0.5 g sodium.

There are a number of salt substitutes available that contain less sodium than regular salt, as a large proportion of the sodium is replaced with potassium. Potassium doesn't have the same effect on blood pressure as sodium, but salt subsitutes based on potassium are not suitable for use by people with heart or kidney disorders, unless under medical supervision.

Sea salt is produced by evaporating sea water and contains iodine and other minerals, which give it a healthier status than ordinary table salt, which is made by mixing rock salt with magnesium carbonate. However, the sodium levels in both are the same.

Reducing the amount of salt you add to food in cooking and at table will help cut your sodium intake, but its more effective to cut down on foods to which salt is already added, such as crisps, sauces, pickles, takeaways, salted meats and so on. Tastebuds slowly become accustomed to using less salt and after a time you will probably find that you become very sensitive to highly salted foods. Experiment with different ways of flavouring food, and choose lightly salted or low-salt versions of products such as bacon or butter.

Sugar

Current government health recommendations say we should all cut down on the amount of sugar we eat. This isn't because sugar is particularly fattening – it contains 3.75 calories per gram, compared to fat at 9 calories per gram and protein at 4 calories per gram. The problem is not really with table sugar. In fact, we are adding less sugar to cereals, drinks and desserts than we used to.

However, we are eating more sugar in processed foods than ever before; at least half the sugar in our diet comes from foods like biscuits, cakes, sweets and soft drinks. For example, a 330 ml can of non-diet cola contains 35 grams of sugar, a 25 grams (1 ounce) portion of sugar-coated cereal contains 10 grams of sugar, and a Mars bar 45 grams of sugar.

Sugars and starches are both forms of carbohydrate. Sugars are often described as simple carbohydrates and starches as complex carbohydrates. Although they have different structures, both provide the same number of calories, gram for gram.

The proper name for common table sugar is sucrose; the sugar in fruit and vegetables is known as fructose or fruit sugar, and the sugar in milk is called lactose. The sugars that are considered to be of least value from a nutritional point of view are those that arent locked into food in some way. Sometimes described as non-milk extrinsic (NME) sugars, these include table sugar, honey and jam.

Sugar is commonly described as containing empty calories, because it provides energy but no nutrients. So to maintain a healthy weight and eat well, we are advised to obtain energy from foods that also provide us with other nutrients.

Yet there may be more aspects to the slimming and sugar story. Some experts even believe that a little sugar can actually help you to slim. For example, dietary surveys have shown that people who get fewer calories from fats tend to get more calories from sugar, and vice versa. This is often referred to as the fat-sugar see-saw. Given that current healthy-eating guidelines are based on reducing fat, some experts feel that advice to eat less fat *and* less sugar may be difficult to follow. And, if eating sugar leads to higher intakes of fat, it's bad news in terms of heart disease and obesity.

Sugar and fat both increase the energy density of a meal but also make food taste really good, so its easier to overeat on these foods without realizing it, as anyone tempted by cream cakes will know! It is for this reason that some researchers feel that a low-fat diet would be more acceptable, tastier and easier to maintain if the fat were replaced with a mixture of calories derived from starch and sugar.

In terms of everyday healthy eating, the conclusion seems to be that sugar and sugary foods can be included as part of a calorie-controlled diet. But as sugar doesn't provide any other nutrients, if you eat too much of it you won't leave many calories for nutritious foods that are high in vitamins and minerals.

If you find that having something sweet or using sugar on cereal satisfies your appetite and stops you snacking, fine, as long as you count the calories.

Eating lots of sugary foods throughout the day promotes tooth decay, so always eat sugary foods with a meal rather than on their own, and avoid eating high-sugar snacks frequently. Saliva helps to neutralize plaque acid, but it doesn't get time to work if you eat sweet foods regularly.

Foods that are high in sugar also tend to be high in fat and calories. Having the odd teaspoonful of sugar on cereal is fine, but regularly eating sugar-containing foods such as chocolates, biscuits and cakes means your fat intake will also be high and you won't slim as efficiently as you'd like to.

Alcohol

Most of us enjoy a drink now and again. Even if you don't drink very much, the chances are you'll indulge at Christmas, weddings or parties. The trouble is, while a few drinks may make the party go with a swing, if you get too carried away you'll wake up with a very weighty conscience. The important thing is to be able to enjoy a drink without damaging your dieting efforts.

First, let's look at how alcohol can affect your diet. You may be thinking that a few glasses of wine can't make that much difference. But alcohol is a hidden enemy: it can sabotage your good intentions in several different ways.

- Alcohol is packed with calories. A small glass of wine can cost you the same as a couple of biscuits, and although spirits can seem quite reasonable, mixers like orange juice and cola can be full of calories too. Choose one that's low in calories or calorie-free.
- The calories in alcohol are empty, that is they contain no nutritional value at all. What a waste of your precious calorie quota! If you cut back on your food intake to save calories for alcoholic drinks you'll miss out on the essential nutrients and vitamins you need to stay healthy.
- Alcohol has the effect of lowering your blood-sugar level. That's why diabetics always have to monitor their alcohol intake very carefully.
- Alcohol weakens your self-control. After a few drinks, its easy to throw caution to the winds and indulge in all those goodies youve been denying yourself. And once you've started eating, you won't know when to stop. What's more, alcohol dulls your tastebuds so you won't even enjoy the food you eat to the full.
- It's a myth that a drink will cheer you up. If you're feeling down, you'll end up even more miserable.
- Alcohol is addictive. One glass can so easily lead to another and another.
- Too much booze leaves you looking red-eyed and blotchy – hardly an incentive to keep up the good work towards the new-look you.

- And then there's the morning after. It's hard to muster up your will-power with a muzzy head. And who wants to exercise with an upset tum? If you have overdone it, don't take the 'hair of the dog'; listen to your body and stay off alcohol for at least 48 hours. Remember, the main cause of a hangover after a night's drinking is dehydration, so try to drink lots of water before going to bed.

Understanding how alcohol affects your body may stop you reaching for that one glass too many. Alcohol is rapidly absorbed into the bloodstream. Within a very short space of time, its on its way to the liver to be processed, so the body can get rid of it. It takes about an hour for the system to rid the body of one unit of alcohol.

If you drink more than this, the excess alcohol will be pumped around your system while it waits for its turn to be processed. In the short term, the alcohol in your bloodstream will give you that light-headed feeling; but if you regularly have high concentrations of alcohol in your blood, it will start to affect your health.

The concentration of alcohol in your blood depends on several factors, including whether you've eaten; your height, weight and age; whether or not you're used to drinking alcohol, and your sex. Research shows that women are more easily affected by alcohol than men, feel the effects for longer and are more at risk of liver damage through heavy drinking. Experts believe this is partly because women's bodies are generally smaller than men's and contain more fat and less water. Alcohol is distributed in the body's water, so when a woman drinks, the alcohol is more concentrated in her system.

There is some evidence that a low-to-moderate consumption of wine can reduce the risk of premature death from illnesses such as heart disease. The reasons for this are not clear, but one possible explanation is that red wine may contain antioxidants and flavonoids, which are thought to prevent coronary heart disease and some forms of cancer. Studies show the opposite to be true of spirits, and beer is thought to have no significant effect on life expectancy. But, whatever the individual properties of your favourite tipple, it makes sense – for both your health and your diet – to keep your alcohol consumption in check.

Two ways to slim

Which is best for slimming, a low-fat diet or a calorie-controlled diet? Broadly speaking, the answer is that they are both a way of measuring the same thing: ensuring that you take in less energy than you expend, and therefore that you will lose weight.

As we've already seen, keeping your fat intake low is good for health reasons. A low-fat diet is likely to be lower in calories than a high-fat diet, because fat is so calorie-dense and because it is harder to overeat on low-fat foods. A calorie-controlled diet, on the other hand, need not be low in fat. (You would probably lose weight by eating only 1000 calories' worth of butter a day, but this is *not* recommended!)

A healthy slimming diet, therefore, should always be low in fat, as are all those recommended by *Slimming*. High-calorie foods tend to be high in fat, so counting calories is one way to keep an eye on fat intake. In the same way, counting fat grams or fat units (see below) is a good way of controlling overall calorie intake.

The main rule for successful slimming is to decide whether to count fat or calories and then to stick to that method. Don't mix and match by counting some foods in calories and some in fat.

Counting calories

Counting calories is the easiest, sure-fire way to lose weight – and keep it off. Calories represent the amount of energy in food and the amount of energy we burn up. The average woman needs around 2000 calories from food each day just to maintain her weight. The heavier and more active you are, the more you burn up. It couldn't be simpler: if you eat fewer calories than your body uses, you'll lose weight, and once you've reached your target weight, if you stick to the number of calories that's right for you, you'll stay there.

Foods vary in their calorie value according to their fat, protein, carbohydrate and alcohol content:

- Fats contain 9 calories per gram.
- Carbohydrates contain 3.75 calories per gram.
- Proteins contain 4 calories per gram.
- Alcohol contains 7 calories per gram.

Reducing your calorie intake can be achieved most easily by cutting down on foods high in fat. In contrast, foods high in carbohydrates (such as bread, pasta and rice) are quite low in calories and should be included in a slimming diet. For a comprehensive list of more than 18,000 calorie-counted foods, look out for *Slimming's Your Greatest Guide to Calories*, which is available from supermarkets and large newsagents, price £1.95.

Many packaged foods have nutrition information on their labels. Values for the energy (calorie) content of food may be given in:

- kilocalories (kcal) – another term for calories – or
- kilojoules (kJ) – the metric measure of energy. One kcal equals 4.2 kJ.

Counting fat

The experts say that no more than a third of our energy should come from fat. In practice, this means that an average woman who consumes 2000 calories a day should eat no more than 65 grams of fat a day. It's therefore possible to lose weight by restricting the number of grams of fat you eat. A woman who is following a diet of 1000 calories a day, for example, should aim for a maximum of 40 grams of fat a day.

Because it is not always easy to know precisely how much fat there is in foods, *Slimming* invented the Fat Unit System. This system counts all the fat in foods you will incorporate in your diet and leaves you free to eat as much fruit and veg as you like.

Slimming invented the Fat Unit System more than fifteen years ago and since then thousands of slimmers have achieved success with it. Basically, it's a low-fat, high-carbohydrate diet that you can adapt to suit your tastes and lifestyle. With this system, you control the amount of fat you eat, and it gives you more freedom than counting calories because there are hundreds of foods you can eat without restriction. This system is more than just a diet: it provides a healthier way to eat – for life.

We've given thousands of foods a value that corresponds to the amount of fat they contain. We have called this a fat unit value. The higher the fat unit value of a food, the more fat it contains. To control your fat intake, all you have to do is count the number of fat units you eat each day. You'll never go hungry, as there are hundreds of foods that are virtually fat-free. You can eat as many of these as you like. We recommend that, to lose weight, you should eat between seven and ten fat units a day (this represents between 25 grams and 30 grams (about an ounce) of fat a day). *Slimming's The Complete Fat Unit Counter* lists the fat unit values of thousands of foods, including both basic foods and manufacturers' products.

How to calculate your energy needs

How active are you? Put a tick beside whichever of the following best describes you:

- **Inactive**
  Exceptionally inactive with no sport or active leisure pursuits. Spends very little time on household chores. Doesn't stand or move about for more than about three hours a day.

- **Average**
  A lifestyle representative of most British adults: a fairly sedentary occupation and little strenuous activity in the home, with occasional sporting activity.

- **Active**
  More active than average because of a manual occupation, regular strenuous leisure pursuits or a significant amount of time spent walking or cycling.

Many overweight people think they have a slower metabolism and therefore burn up fewer calories than thin people. But scientists have proved the opposite – most overweight people have a higher metabolic rate than thin people, because it takes more energy to move their excess weight about.

　　The calorie expenditure tables below are a useful guide to the estimated number of calories you burn up each day, depending on your weight and activity level. They may well surprise you. Few 16-stone (100-kilo) women would believe their likely energy expenditure is over 2500 calories a day, and that even a moderate diet of 1500 calories a day would cause a weight loss of about 2 pounds (a kilo) a week, since a pound (455 grams) of fat is equivalent to about 3500 calories.

Even if you weigh only 9 stone 6 pounds (60 kilos) and are inactive, you still need 1730 calories just to maintain that weight. So if you think you're only eating 1000 calories a day and cannot understand why you're not losing weight, the most likely explanation is that you're not weighing or recording what you're eating accurately enough.

Calorie expenditure for women
(calories per day)

Body weight

St	lb	Kg	Inactive	Average	Active
7	1	45	1570	1820	2060
7	12	50	1630	1880	2130
8	9	55	1680	1940	2190
9	6	60	1730	2000	2260
10	3	65	1780	2060	2330
11	0	70	1830	2120	2400
11	11	75	1890	2180	2465
12	8	80	1950	2250	2550
13	5	85	2000	2310	2620
14	2	90	2050	2370	2690
14	13	95	2110	2430	2750
15	10	100	2160	2490	2820
16	7	105	2210	2550	2890
17	4	110	2260	2610	2960
18	1	115	2310	2670	3030
18	12	120	2370	2730	3090
19	9	125	2420	2790	3160

Calorie expenditure for men
(calories per day)

Body weight

St	lb	Kg	Inactive	Average	Active
9	6	60	2030	2340	2650
10	3	65	2100	2430	2750
11	0	70	2180	2510	2850
11	11	75	2250	2600	2950
12	8	80	2330	2690	3040
13	5	85	2400	2770	3140
14	2	90	2480	2860	3240
14	13	95	2550	2940	3340
15	10	100	2630	3030	3430
16	7	105	2700	3120	3530
17	4	110	2780	3200	3630
18	1	115	2850	3290	3730
18	12	120	2920	3370	3820
19	9	125	3000	3460	3920

If you're already at your ideal weight, but don't trust yourself to eat sensibly, you can use our chart to work out the number of calories you need each day. If your weight isn't listed, go to the two weights it falls between to get an average of the calorie expenditure values given.

For example, if you are a woman who weighs 10 stone 7 pounds (67 kilos) and your activity level is average, your estimated calorie expenditure will be around 2060 (the value given for 10 stone 3) plus 2120 (the value given for 11 stone) divided by 2 = 2090 calories per day. So, as long as your calorie intake doesn't exceed that number, you won't put on any more weight.

If you're aiming to lose weight, you'll need to eat fewer

calories than your body burns up. However, often when you begin eating less, your body tries to conserve energy by slowing down the metabolism, so you will in fact burn up fewer calories than stated here. To account for this and bearing in mind the amount of weight you want to lose, these are the calorie intakes we recommend to achieve an effective weight loss of about 2lb per week:

- less than a stone (6 kilos) to lose: 1000 calories a day
- between 1and 3 stone (6–20 kilos) to lose: 1250 calories a day
- more than 3 stone (20 kilos) to lose: 1500 calories a day.

What weight should you be?

To stay fit and healthy, you should weigh the right amount for your height. Being overweight means you are more likely to suffer from diabetes, heart disease, high blood pressure, certain cancers, gallstones and joint and back problems. But it's also unhealthy to be underweight, as you may not be eating enough food to provide all the nutrients needed for good health.

Look at the chart on page 74 to see if you are a suitable weight for your height. This chart applies to adult men and women, but is not suitable for assessing the weight of children or teenagers, pregnant women or sportspeople who have a high proportion of muscle.

The chart is based on the calculation of the BMI (body mass index). You can calculate your own BMI by dividing your weight in kilograms by your height in metres squared. Ideally, your BMI should be between 20 and 25.

- If you are Underweight, you may need to eat more in order to gain weight. Choose nourishing foods instead of fatty and sugary snacks.

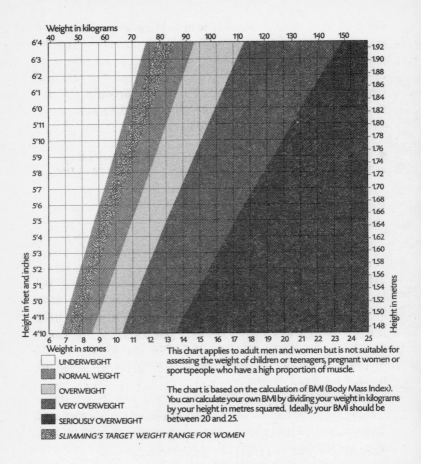

Weight in kilograms

UNDERWEIGHT

NORMAL WEIGHT

OVERWEIGHT

VERY OVERWEIGHT

SERIOUSLY OVERWEIGHT

SLIMMING'S TARGET WEIGHT RANGE FOR WOMEN

This chart applies to adult men and women but is not suitable for assessing the weight of children or teenagers, pregnant women or sportspeople who have a high proportion of muscle.

The chart is based on the calculation of BMI (Body Mass Index). You can calculate your own BMI by dividing your weight in kilograms by your height in metres squared. Ideally, your BMI should be between 20 and 25.

- If you are Normal Weight, try to keep your weight steady and don't be tempted to aim for the underweight category. If your weight has been gradually increasing within this range, now is the time to take action so you don't become overweight. Within the normal weight range, you will see a separate area has been highlighted.

This area is *Slimming*'s target weight range for women (see below for details).

- If you are **overweight**, avoid gaining weight. Aim to lose weight at a rate of 1–2 pounds (½–1 kilo) per week.

- If you are **very overweight**, it's essential that you lose weight. Even small losses will benefit your health.

- If you are **seriously overweight**, it's absolutely essential that you lose weight, as your health is seriously at risk. You may find it helpful to talk to your doctor.

Find your comfort zone

Slimming has devised its own unique target weight charts (see pages 76 and 77), based on the weights at which people tell us they feel happiest about their size and shape. For women, a weight range is given. For example, if you are 5 foot 6, your target weight is between 9 stone 4 and 10 stone 2. (In the chart on page 74, you will see that *Slimming*'s target weight range for women is in the middle of the 'normal weight' section. The tables overleaf represent target weights equivalent to BMI 21 to 23 for women and a maximum of BMI 25 for men.)

Choose a weight between the two values at which you think you will feel most comfortable. As you get closer to this weight, you may wish to adjust your target.

For men, only a maximum weight is given (looking at the top chart, the maximum ideal weight for men equates to the line dividing the 'normal' and 'overweight' sections.)

Avoid weighing yourself more than once a week; your weight can fluctuate during the day and from day to day. The heights do not include footwear, but the ideal weights include an allowance of 2 to 3 pounds (about 1 kilo) for light clothing.

Target weight chart for women

Weight range (in indoor clothes)					Height (without shoes)		
st	lb	st	lb	kg	ft	in	m
7	2 –	7	12	45.5 – 50.0	4	10	1.47
7	6 –	8	2	47.2 – 51.8	4	11	1.50
7	9 –	8	6	48.6 – 53.6	5	0	1.52
7	13 –	8	10	50.5 – 55.5	5	1	1.55
8	3 –	9	0	52.3 – 57.3	5	2	1.57
8	6 –	9	4	53.6 – 59.1	5	3	1.60
8	10 –	9	8	55.5 – 60.9	5	4	1.63
9	0 –	9	12	57.3 – 62.7	5	5	1.65
9	4 –	10	2	59.1 – 64.5	5	6	1.68
9	8 –	10	6	60.9 – 66.4	5	7	1.70
9	12 –	10	11	62.7 – 68.6	5	8	1.73
10	2 –	11	1	64.5 – 70.5	5	9	1.75
10	6 –	11	6	66.4 – 72.7	5	10	1.78
10	10 –	11	11	68.2 – 75.0	5	11	1.80
11	0 –	12	1	70.0 – 76.8	6	0	1.93

Why crash dieting isn't the answer

There's no magic formula

Most of us have tried to diet at some stage in our lives and most will admit to wanting the fastest results possible. Many commercial diet regimes tempt us with the promise of quick results from diet plans that vary from following diets high in protein and low in carbohydrates, to weird food combinations and liquid meal-replacement diets. The choices and conflicting claims are bewildering.

Target weight chart for men

Max weight* (in indoor clothes)			Height (without shoes)		
st	lb	kg	ft	in	m
9	10	61.8	5	2	1.57
10	1	64.1	5	3	1.60
10	5	65.9	5	4	1.63
10	10	68.2	5	5	1.65
11	1	70.5	5	6	1.68
11	5	72.3	5	7	1.70
11	10	74.5	5	8	1.73
12	1	76.8	5	9	1.75
12	6	79.1	5	10	1.78
12	11	81.4	5	11	1.80
13	2	83.6	6	0	1.83
13	7	85.9	6	1	1.85
13	12	88.2	6	2	1.88
14	4	90.9	6	3	1.90
14	9	93.2	6	4	1.93

* Final waist measurement should be less than hip measurement.

Slimming's philosophy has nothing in common with these irrational diets; it is based on healthy eating and wholesome foods. There is no special food, no magic combination of foods and no formula that increases weight loss. For example, grapefruit does not burn calories, and the order in which foods are consumed does not affect a person's weight.

The most effective way to lose weight is to eat a variety of nutritious, high-carbohydrate, low-fat foods that overall contain fewer calories than you need, and to take more exercise. You should be aiming at a weight loss of between 1 and 2 pounds (450 to 900 grams) a week. If you lose weight any faster than this, you may be at risk of losing muscle tissue as well as fat, which is not good for your general health and will eventually slow down your weight loss even further.

The following section gives some more reasons why crash dieting is a bad idea.

Fad diets are unsociable, boring and expensive

The constant evolution of dubious fad or crash diets occurs because their success rate is low and most are boring, unsociable or too expensive. Each year in the UK, millions of pounds are spent on meal replacements and formula diets, designed to replace normal eating with a calorie-controlled drink, mix, bar or rehydrated meal.

Such regimes can seem successful in the initial stages of a diet (particularly if someone is extremely overweight) but they do not help to educate slimmers about the importance of sensible, healthy eating, and make it more likely the weight won't stay off. In fact, those who lose weight on faddy regimes have a 95 per cent chance of putting the weight back on in the first year. As it can take several months to reach a target weight, a diet must be palatable and enjoyable enough to be followed for long periods.

If you enjoy food, it's unlikely you'll keep to a regime where tasty meals are replaced with bland shakes, bars or potions. It's cheaper and tastier to lose weight by altering your everyday foods than by replacing them with fad diet products.

Fad diets can also ruin your social life. It won't be long before you tire of turning down every offer of a meal out or trip to the pub. Effective diets must allow an occasional meal out or treat. Otherwise, they just won't last.

You always put the weight back on after a crash diet

The sequence of losing and regaining weight is probably depressingly familiar to many crash dieters. This eternal cycle has been appropriately labelled 'yo-yo dieting'. About 95 per cent of crash dieters regain their weight, which is hardly surprising when you think how difficult it is to stick to a regime that requires virtual starvation, or replaces tasty everyday meals with synthetic drinks and rehydrated meals. The metabolic effects of such regimes make them impossible to consider as a long-term solution to a weight problem.

In the past, yo-yo dieting has been said to increase a dieter's resistance to weight loss, but there is no evidence to support this. However, there is the possibility that yo-yo dieting may increase the risk of certain diseases such as diabetes, high blood pressure and coronary heart disease. It is therefore vital that a weight loss regime should change your eating habits for life, so preventing future weight gain or yo-yo dieting.

Once you've lost weight, you need to adapt your eating habits to supply the correct number of calories for your new body weight: with less weight to carry, your body needs fewer calories.

Crash diets makes you feel tired, hungry and moody

It's tempting to think that the quickest way to lose weight is by starvation on a crash diet. Those of you who have tried this will probably be familiar with the resultant feelings of extreme hunger, irritation, depression, tiredness and cravings. We have all heard of someone who has lost 10 pounds (4.5 kilos) in a week on a crash diet, but what most of us don't realize is that the weight lost is mostly fluid, not fat.

When the body is deprived of calories, the blood sugar level drops and an instant store of energy called glycogen (a type of natural sugar) is mobilized from the liver and muscles. Glycogen contains nearly three parts water, and when it's burned up to provide energy, the water is excreted in urine: this accounts for most of the weight loss in the first few days of dieting.

When the glycogen stores have run out, weight loss slows down, which can be disheartening. Deprived of glycogen, the body also slows down, causing tiredness, depression and irritability – all common complaints among crash dieters. Glycogen also controls the appetite; low stores will trigger extreme hunger. The result is that most crash dieters succeed in losing weight, but soon give in to acute hunger pangs, causing the pounds (and guilt) to quickly reappear.

Crash dieting lowers your metabolic rate

When the body is deprived of adequate calories, it uses its own stores of glycogen, fat and protein to maintain body functions. This affects our metabolic rate (a measure of the amount of energy we burn up). Our bodies store up to about one day's worth of energy in the form of glycogen, and once this reserve has been used up, the body will call upon its other stores. But it will not exclusively use fat tissue: between 14 and 25 per cent of the total weight loss will be lean tissue, i.e. muscle. Muscle cells are made up of proteins and they require lots of energy to function, whereas fat cells need very little.

If we fast or crash diet, our bodies start to break down muscle tissue as well as fat, in order to provide energy. This decrease in muscle mass results in a lowering of the metabolic rate: an in-built survival mechanism that comes into operation when the body thinks it's being starved. As a result of this lowered metabolic rate, we need to eat fewer calories just to match the reduced number of calories we will now burn up and enable us to maintain our weight.

Prompting the survival mechanism not only makes it more difficult to lose weight, but increases the chances of regaining weight. A slow but steady weight loss (of between 1 and 2 pounds [450 to 900 grams] a week) minimizes the loss of lean tissue (muscles), and so helps to maintain the metabolic rate at its normal level. Following a sensible diet of between 1000 and 1750 calories a day therefore makes it less likely that weight will be regained.

In an average person, about 75 per cent of total energy expenditure is used to operate the body's basic activities, such as breathing, heartbeat and maintaining body temperature. This is called the body's basal metabolic rate (BMR) and is partly determined by body composition, i.e. the amounts of lean tissue and body fat you have. This means that exercise, if carried out on a regular basis, is also a good way to increase your BMR, as it increases the muscle mass of the body.

A further 10 per cent of your total calorie expenditure is needed to digest food and the remaining 15 per cent accounts for all of your other activities, including physical exercise.

Crash diets can be dangerous

The reported hazards of fasting or very low-calorie diets (VLCDs) – those under 600 calories a day – include nausea, dizziness, dehydration, fatigue, bad breath, ketosis (an excess of certain acids in the blood, one symptom is that the breath smells of acetone), increased uric acid levels in the blood, and, in rare cases, heart, kidney or liver failure. These conditions can all be attributed to the changes in metabolism that occur when the body is deprived of adequate fuel.

The brain needs a constant supply of glucose in order to operate, and when you crash diet, glucose has to be taken from other reserves. A sudden drop in blood glucose levels causes confusion and changes in behaviour (like those experienced by diabetes sufferers). Government recommendations state that VLCDs should only be used by obese people whose excess weight puts their health at risk. Also, they should only be used under the strict supervision of a doctor, and when a traditional, calorie-restricted diet has failed.

4

Recipes for year-round body confidence

Make time for breakfast

Research shows that starting the day with a healthy, filling breakfast is one of the most powerful allies in a slimming campaign, and it's certainly true that many successful slimmers featured in *Slimming* report that making time for breakfast was one of the most valuable changes they made to their eating habits when they started to lose weight.

Many people who are 'too busy' for breakfast or 'can't face food first thing' find that by mid-morning they are extremely hungry and are likely to fill up on snacks like biscuits or cakes. Thinking that you can save calories by skipping breakfast is a false economy. Studies have proved that people who eat breakfast actually tend to consume fewer calories over the whole day than those who do not.

Breakfast does not have to be an elaborate meal, and you needn't eat it the moment you leap out of bed. But if you start the day with breakfast it is likely that you will have more energy throughout the day, be less likely to snack, and find your other meals more satisfying.

So, if you haven't got the breakfast habit, why not try some of these easy and tasty ideas? If you are stuck in a cereal rut, there are some imaginative alternatives. They all provide around 200 calories.

Quantities

- The conversions given in the lists of ingredients are approximate.
- Choose either metric or imperial measures in any one recipe.
- The rough metric equivalents for spoon measures are:

2.5 ml	=	½ tsp
5 ml	=	1 tsp
10 ml	=	2 tsp
15 ml	=	1 tbsp
20 ml	=	4 tsp
30 ml	=	2 tbsp
45 ml	=	3 tbsp
60 ml	=	4 tbsp
90 ml	=	6 tbsp

Toasted pancake with syrup

2 Scotch pancakes, toasted
2 level tsp maple syrup

Toast, orange juice and yogurt

1 medium slice (35 g/1¼ oz) wholemeal bread, toasted
1 level tsp low-fat spread
150 ml/¼ pint unsweetened orange juice
125 g/4½ oz pot diet yogurt

Crunchy yogurt and fruit

150 g/5 oz pot low-fat natural yogurt
15 g/½ oz muesli, with no added sugar
1 small banana, sliced

Bacon and tomato roll and a satsuma

1 50 g/2 oz wholemeal bread roll
1 rasher lean back bacon, well grilled
1 tomato, grilled
1 level tbsp brown sauce or tomato ketchup
1 satsuma

Porridge with raisins and honey

25 g/1 oz porridge oats
150 ml/¼ pint skimmed milk
1 level tbsp raisins
1 level tsp honey

Weetabix cereal

2 Weetabix biscuits
150 ml/¼ pint skimmed milk
1 level tsp sugar

Croissant and jam

1 40 g/1½ oz croissant
2 level tsp jam

Egg on toast and a satsuma

1 medium egg, poached or boiled
1 medium (35 g/1¼ oz) slice wholemeal bread, toasted
1 level tsp low-fat spread
1 satsuma

Greek yogurt and honey

115 g/4 oz Greek-style yogurt
1 level tsp honey

Crumpet and orange juice

1 40 g/1¼ oz crumpet
1 level tsp low-fat spread
¼ pint unsweetened orange juice

English breakfast

1 low-fat pork sausage, grilled
1 rasher lean back bacon (25 g/1 oz raw weight), grilled
1 tomato, grilled

Bran cereal and yogurt

25 g/1 oz bran cereal
150 ml ¼ pint skimmed milk
125 g/4½ oz pot diet yogurt

Muffin and honey

1 65 g/2½ oz muffin, toasted
2 level tsp low-fat spread
2 level tsp honey

Grapefruit, toast and preserves

½ grapefruit
1 medium (35 g/1¼ oz) slice wholemeal bread, toasted
1 level tsp low-fat spread
1 level tsp jam or marmalade

Fresh ideas for Spring

Springtime paella

SERVES 4

410 calories per serving
3½ fat units per serving
10 g fat per serving
Preparation time: 30 minutes
Cooking time: 45 minutes

four 50 g/2 oz chicken drumsticks, skin removed
1 level tsp Cajun seasoning
4 tsp oil
175 g/6 oz mussels
150 ml/¼ pint dry white wine
3 sprigs fresh thyme
1 small onion, thinly sliced

2 cloves of garlic, finely chopped
35 g/1¼ oz chorizo sausage, sliced
1 red pepper, deseeded and diced
pinch of saffron
pinch of paprika
200 g/7 oz long-grain rice
pinch of salt
850 ml/1½ pints fresh chicken stock
150 g/5 oz tiger prawns
50 g/2 oz crab sticks
50 g/2 oz peas
freshly ground black pepper

1 Preheat the oven to 190°C/375°F/gas mark 5. Make several slits in each drumstick with a sharp knife and place in an ovenproof dish, then sprinkle with Cajun seasoning. Brush with half the oil and bake for 35 minutes.
2 Meanwhile, clean the mussels and remove any beards. Place the wine and thyme in a pan, bring to the boil and add the mussels. Cover with a tight-fitting lid and steam for a few minutes until the shells open.
3 Discard any unopened shells, then drain the open mussels, reserving the liquid, and set on one side.
4 Heat the remaining oil in a large non-stick pan and sauté the onion and garlic for 3 to 4 minutes until softened. Add the sausage and red pepper and cook for a further 3 minutes.
5 Add the saffron and paprika to the pan, cook for a further minute, then stir in the rice and a pinch of salt. Cook for a few minutes more, then stir in the stock and bring to the boil.
6 Add the mussels and reserved liquid together with the prawns, crab sticks and peas. Season to taste, then simmer gently for 25 minutes, stirring occasionally.

Bacon and tomato risotto

SERVES 4

290 calories per serving
5½ fat units per serving
16 g fat per serving
Preparation time: 20 minutes
Cooking time: 35 minutes

115 g/4 oz lean back bacon
4 tsp oil
1 small onion, roughly chopped
2 cloves garlic, finely chopped
150 g/5 oz risotto or arborio rice
1 tsp dried thyme
200 ml/7 fl oz dry white wine
275 ml/½ pint fresh vegetable stock
2 medium tomatoes, roughly chopped
115 g/4 oz yellow or brown oyster mushrooms, quartered
4 spring onions, roughly chopped
3 tbsp Parmesan cheese, grated
freshly ground black pepper
1 level tbsp fresh parsley, chopped

1 Grill the bacon and cut into bite-sized pieces. Heat the oil in a non-stick pan and sauté the onion and garlic for 4 to 5 minutes until a light golden brown.
2 Add the rice and thyme to the pan. Cook for 3 minutes, stirring occasionally, add the wine and stock, then bring to the boil, reduce the heat and simmer gently for 15 minutes.
3 Add the bacon, tomatoes, mushrooms and spring onions, and cook for 5 minutes.
4 Transfer to a serving plate and sprinkle with Parmesan cheese. Season with black pepper and serve garnished with chopped parsley.

Stuffed pepper

SERVES 1

300 calories per serving
4½ fat units per serving
13 g fat per serving
Preparation time: 10 minutes
Cooking time: 40 minutes

1 medium red pepper
25 g/1 oz couscous
50 g/2 oz courgettes, chopped
1 or 2 spring onions, trimmed and chopped
1 tsp oil
25 g/1 oz frozen or fresh peas
pinch of ground cinnamon
15 g/½ oz cashew nuts
2 level tsp raisins
salt and freshly ground pepper

1 Preheat the oven to 190°C/375°F/gas mark 5. Cut the top off the pepper and remove the seeds and pith. Cook the couscous according to the packet instructions, then drain thoroughly. Fry the courgettes and spring onions in the oil until soft. Cook the peas, then drain.
2 Mix all the ingredients together, season, and fill the pepper.
3 Stand the pepper in an ovenproof dish and add a little water to the bottom of the dish. Bake for 40 minutes.

Stir-fried spring vegetables

SERVES 2

165 calories per serving
3½ fat units per serving
10 g fat per serving
Preparation time: 10 minutes
Cooking time: 5 minutes

1 tbsp olive oil
1.25cm/½ inch piece fresh ginger, grated
1 clove garlic, crushed
75 g/3 oz baby carrots, trimmed
50 g/2 oz French beans, trimmed
75 g/3 oz baby courgettes, halved lengthways
50 g/2 oz mangetout or sugar-snap peas, trimmed
50 g/2 oz baby corn-cobs, halved lengthways
2 spring onions, shredded
75 g/3 oz bean sprouts
freshly ground black pepper
1 tsp sesame oil

Sauce:
4 tsp sherry
4 tsp soy sauce
1 level tsp thin honey

1 Combine the sauce ingredients.
2 Heat the oil in a large non-stick pan. Then add the ginger, garlic, carrots, and French beans, and stir-fry for 2 minutes. Add the remaining vegetables and stir-fry for a further 2 minutes.
3 Season with freshly ground black pepper and sprinkle with sesame oil. Serve immediately, mixed with the sauce.

Tarragon and avocado-topped tuna

SERVES 4

310 calories per serving
5 fat units per serving
14 g fat per serving
Preparation and marinating time: 40 minutes
Grilling time: 15 minutes

four 150 g/5 oz fresh tuna steaks
salt and freshly ground black pepper
1 tbsp fresh tarragon
2 tbsp lemon juice
1 tbsp olive oil
1 ripe medium avocado
2 tbsp reduced-fat mayonnaise
2 tbsp fat-free fromage frais
few drops of Tabasco sauce
slices of lemon, to garnish

1 Place the tuna in an ovenproof dish and season with salt and pepper. Sprinkle with the olive oil and 2 tsp of the tarragon and 1 tbsp of the lemon juice. Marinate for 30 minutes.
2 Meanwhile, put the avocado flesh in a food processor with the rest of the lemon juice and the mayonnaise and fromage frais and blend until smooth. Season with Tabasco sauce, stir in the remaining tarragon and chill until required.
3 Put the tuna on a foil-covered tray and grill for six minutes each side. Top with the avocado sauce and garnish with the lemon slices.

Roasted rich tomato soup

SERVES 4

175 calories per serving
3 fat units per serving
9 g fat per serving
Preparation time: 30 minutes
Cooking time: 1 hour 15 minutes

1.3 kg/3 lb plum tomatoes
2 tbsp extra virgin olive oil
1 tsp sea salt
2 tbsp caster sugar
1 red chilli (optional)
1 small onion
1 clove garlic
4 tsp sun-dried tomato paste
2 tbsp lime juice
salt and freshly ground black pepper

1 Cut the tomatoes in half lengthways, scoop out the seeds and discard. Cover a baking tray with foil and lightly grease with 2 tsp of the oil.

2 Lay the tomatoes on the foil, cut side upwards, and sprinkle with another 2 tsp of oil, the sea salt and the caster sugar. Add the chilli, if using, and cook at 180°C/350°F/gas mark 4 for 40 minutes. Remove the chilli after 20 minutes if used.

3 Heat the remaining oil in a non-stick pan and sauté the finely chopped onion and garlic for 6 to 7 minutes until lightly golden. Stir in the tomato paste, the tomatoes and any juice from the tray, together with 575 ml/1 pint water. Bring to the boil.

4 Reduce the heat and simmer for 15 minutes. Cool slightly, then purée until smooth. Stir in the lime juice and add salt and pepper to taste. Serve with crusty bread (count calories separately).

Honey banana fool

SERVES 6

235 calories per serving
3 fat units per serving
8 g fat per serving
Preparation time: 20 minutes
Chilling time: 2 hours

6 tbsp honey
3 ripe medium bananas
juice of one lemon
225 g/8 oz fromage frais, 8 per cent fat
115 g/4 oz Greek-style yogurt
40 g/1½ oz fructose

To decorate:
15 g/½ oz toasted desiccated coconut
lemon zest
fresh mint sprigs

1 Heat the honey until runny and divide between six goblet glasses. Chill while the fool is made.
2 Meanwhile, mash up the bananas with a fork until smooth and mix in the lemon juice. Cream the fromage frais, yogurt and fructose together until smooth. Chill this until the honey has set.
3 Spoon the fool mixture on to the honey and serve sprinkled with the coconut, lemon zest and fresh mint.

Tropical fruit cups

SERVES 6

155 calories per serving
1½ fat units per serving
4 g fat per serving
Preparation time: 20 minutes
Chilling time: 1 hour (minimum)

500 g/1 lb pack frozen red fruits mixture,
defrosted and drained
50 g/2 oz fructose
200 g/7 oz carton reduced-fat crème fraîche
200 g/7 oz reduced-fat strawberry fromage frais
200 g/7 oz pack ready-prepared mango slices
sprinkling of ground cinnamon

1 Reserve some of the red fruits mixture for decoration and combine the remainder with the fructose. Mix the reduced-fat crème fraîche and fromage frais together. Halve the mango slices.
2 Take six ramekins and put a spoonful of the red fruits mixture into the base of each. Cover with mango slices, then add some of the crème fraîche and fromage frais mixture. Sprinkle with cinnamon, then repeat the layers.
3 Chill for at least one hour. Before serving, decorate with the reserved red fruits.

Crème caramel

SERVES 6

200 calories per serving
2 fat units per serving
6 g fat per serving
Preparation time: 15 minutes
Cooking time: 45 minutes

130 g/4½ oz caster sugar
150 ml/¼ pint water
4 medium eggs
575 ml/1 pint semi-skimmed milk
few drops vanilla essence
6 small clementines

1　Preheat the oven to 170°C/325°F/gas mark 3.
2　Put 115 g/4 oz of the sugar in a small non-stick pan with 150 ml/¼ pint water. Heat gently, stirring occasionally, until the sugar has dissolved.
3　Bring to the boil, then simmer until the syrup is golden brown. Remove from the heat, leave for 5 seconds, then pour into 6 small freezer-proof containers and set aside.
4　In a large bowl, whisk the eggs with the remaining sugar. Warm the milk in a pan and add to the bowl. Add the vanilla essence, then strain the mixture into a jug.
5　Pour the custard mixture into the prepared containers and place in a roasting tin. Pour enough hot water into the tin to come half-way up the sides of the containers.
6　Bake for 40 minutes, until the custard is just set.
7　Remove the crème caramels from the tin and leave until cold. Cover with clingfilm and refrigerate for at least 1 hour.
8　Turn out onto individual serving plates. Peel the clementines and arrange the segments around each caramel.

Pineapple and honey upside-down puds

SERVES 6

245 calories per serving
3 fat units per serving
9 g fat per serving
Preparation time: 30 minutes
Cooking time: 25 minutes

1 tsp oil for greasing
227 g/8 oz can pineapple chunks in natural juice
1 level tbsp honey
115 g/4 oz half-fat spread
115 g/4 oz fructose
1 large egg
115 g/4 oz plain flour
1½ level tsp cornflour

1 Preheat the oven to 190°C/375°F/gas mark 5. Lightly grease six small pudding dishes or ramekins, 8 cm (3 inches) in diameter, then place a small circle of grease-proof paper in the base of each.

2 Drain the pineapple, reserving the juice. Divide the pineapple chunks evenly between the dishes and drizzle a little honey over each.

3 Cream the spread and the fructose together until well blended. Add the lightly beaten egg, then carefully fold in the sieved flour.

4 Divide the mixture between the dishes – it should cover the pineapple. Level the surface with a knife, then bake in the oven for 15 to 18 minutes until well-risen, golden brown and firm to touch.

5 Meanwhile, prepare the sauce. Mix the cornflour with the reserved pineapple juice. Heat in a pan, stirring until thickened. Keep warm.

6 Once the puddings are cooked, use a knife to ease around the edge of each, turn them out and serve with the sauce.

Cherry swirls

SERVES 6

180 calories per serving
2 fat units per serving
6 g fat per serving
Preparation time: 20 minutes

275 g/10 oz fat-free fromage frais
200 g/7 oz tub low-calorie black
or red cherry yogurt
150 g/5 oz mascarpone cheese
400 g/14 oz can reduced-sugar black
or red cherry pie filling

1 Mix the fromage frais, yogurt and mascarpone cheese together until smooth and creamy.
2 Purée the cherry pie filling until smooth. Roughly stir half of the purée into the soft cheese.
3 Take six glasses and place some of the purée in each, then top with some of the creamy mixture. Repeat these layers until you run out of the creamy mixture. Drizzle some fruit purée on top and serve.

Chocolate crunch

SERVES 8

250 calories per serving
2½ fat units per serving
6 g fat per serving
Preparation and freezing time: 1 hour 15 minutes

115 g/4 oz ready to eat dried prunes
275 g/10 oz reduced-fat shortcake biscuits
225 g/8 oz reduced-fat chocolate ice cream topping
175 g/6 oz reduced fat crème fraîche

To serve:
a little icing sugar
2 tbsp low-fat, ready to eat custard
25 g/1 oz raspberries/strawberries, sliced

1 Line a 23 cm/9 inch loose-bottomed cake tin with grease-proof paper. Process the prunes and the biscuits in a blender until roughly chopped.
2 Reserving some for decoration, heat the chocolate topping until runny. Add the crème fraîche, prunes and biscuits and stir well.
3 Spoon into the tin and place in the fast-freeze compartment of the freezer for one hour. Slice.
4 Decorate with a dusting of icing sugar, then serve with the strawberries, custard and reserved chocolate topping.

Sunshine menus for Summer

King prawn and bacon salad

SERVES 3

280 calories per serving
18 g fat per serving
6 fat units per serving
Preparation and marinating time: 2 hours 20 minutes
Cooking time: 8 minutes

six 25 g/1 oz rashers lean back bacon
12 king prawns, cooked and peeled
freshly ground black pepper
2 tbsp lemon or lime juice
1 tbsp olive oil
1 small red onion
6 spring onions
1 yellow or red pepper, deseeded
12 cherry tomatoes

Tarragon dressing:
2 tbsp olive oil
2 tbsp lemon juice
salt and freshly ground black pepper
1 tsp Dijon mustard
1 tbsp fresh tarragon, freshly torn
zest of half a lime
zest of half a lemon

1 Cut each bacon rasher in half, wrap around the centre
part of each prawn and place in a non-metallic dish.
Season with pepper and spoon over the lemon or lime

juice and olive oil. Leave to marinate for one to two hours, tossing twice.

2 To make the dressing, mix all the ingredients together and chill until required.

3 Slice the red onion thinly, cut the spring onions and the pepper into thin strips and halve the cherry tomatoes. Place on a serving dish and pour over the dressing.

4 Place the prawns on a foil-covered tray and grill for 4 to 5 minutes, turning once, until the bacon is crispy. Serve on the salad, sprinkled with lemon and lime zest, if required.

Smoked chicken and pear salad

SERVES 4

310 calories per serving
18 g fat per serving
6½ fat units per serving
Preparation time: 45 minutes
Cooking time: 15 minutes

2 tbsp caster sugar
4 medium-sized firm pears
1 tbsp ginger syrup
2 tbsp lemon juice
350 g/12 oz smoked lean chicken
50 g/2 oz cucumber
1 medium-ripe peach or nectarine

Curry dressing:
4 tsp mild curry paste
1 tbsp mango chutney
50 g/2 oz fat-free fromage frais
3 tbsp reduced-fat crème fraîche

To decorate:
115 g/4 oz raspberries
half a tsp pink peppercorns, roughly crushed
half a tsp black peppercorns, coarsely ground
flat-leaf parsley

1 Put 425 ml/ ¾ pint cold water and the caster sugar in a saucepan. Heat gently until the sugar has dissolved and then bring to the boil.
2 Peel the pears, leaving the stalks intact. Place in the pan with the ginger syrup and lemon juice, lower the heat and cook gently for 15 to 20 minutes. Drain and set on one side.
3 Thinly slice the chicken, cucumber and peach or nectarine and arrange on serving plates with the pear.
4 Stir the dressing ingredients until smooth, reserving 4 tsp of the fromage frais to garnish. Pour the dressing over the ingredients on the serving plates.
5 Spoon over the reserved fromage frais and decorate with raspberries, peppercorn and parsley.

Stuffed mushrooms

SERVES 1

300 calories per serving
4½ fat units per serving
13 g fat per serving

175 g/6 oz large open-cap mushrooms
50 g/2 oz lean back bacon rashers
2 spring onions
half a small clove garlic
1 level tsp olive oil

½ level tsp dried mixed herbs
25 g/10 oz wholemeal breadcrumbs
15 g/½ oz reduced-fat Cheddar cheese, grated

1 Preheat oven to 190°C/375°F/gas mark 5. Remove the stems from the mushrooms and chop. Place the mushrooms, underside up, in an ovenproof dish.
2 Chop the bacon, and the spring onions, and crush the garlic. Heat the oil in a small pan and cook the bacon, onions, garlic and mushroom stems until the bacon is cooked.
3 Stir in the herbs and breadcrumbs, then pile the mixture into the mushroom caps. Sprinkle the cheese on top. Pour a little water into the base of the dish to a level of about 6 mm (¼ inch). Bake for about 20 minutes.

Mozzarella salad with avocado salsa

SERVES 6

225 calories per serving
12 g fat per serving
4½ fat units per serving
Preparation time: 30 minutes
Chilling time: 1 hour

175 g/6 oz reduced-fat mozzarella cheese, thinly sliced
3 beef tomatoes, thinly sliced
2 medium-sized peaches or nectarines, thinly sliced
12 cherry tomatoes
freshly ground black pepper
sprigs of fresh basil
8 green olives

Avocado salsa:
4 cm/2 in piece cucumber, diced
1 small red or yellow pepper, deseeded and diced
50 g/2 oz red onion, finely chopped
1 small ripe avocado, diced
2 tbsp lime juice
2 tbsp virgin olive oil
2 tbsp red pesto

1 To make the salsa, mix together the cucumber, pepper, onion and garlic. Toss in the avocado and immediately mix in the lime juice and olive oil. Lightly toss in the red pesto and chill until required.
2 Arrange the cheese, peaches and large tomatoes on a serving plate in a layered pattern. Season with pepper, basil sprigs and olives. Serve with a spoonful of the salsa per portion.

Honeyed duck with fresh berries

SERVES 4

250 calories per serving
12 g fat per serving
4 fat units per serving
Preparation time: 2½ hours
Cooking time: 35 minutes

two 175 g/6 oz duck breasts, skinned
2 tbsp thin honey
1 tsp Chinese five-spice powder
½ tsp salt
2 tbsp olive oil
1 medium-sized ripe mango
115 g/4 oz strawberries or raspberries (optional)

lettuce (as much as you like)
50 g/2 oz redcurrants
6 tbsp raspberry vinegar
1 tsp black pepper, coarsely ground
fresh mint to garnish

1 Wash and dry the duck and make several slits in each breast. Blend together the honey, five-spice powder, salt and oil and pour evenly over the duck. Leave to marinate for at least two hours, or overnight.

2 Preheat the oven to 200°C/400°F/gas mark 6. Transfer the duck to a wire rack and bake for 30 minutes, until the meat is tender and crispy on the outside. Allow to cool slightly, then slice thinly.

3 Peel and thinly slice the mango, slice the strawberries or raspberries, if used, and toss together with the lettuce and redcurrants in the raspberry vinegar. Place the salad on a serving dish, with the warm sliced duck on top. Sprinkle with pepper and decorate with fresh mint.

Chicken paupiettes with apricot

SERVES 2

340 calories per serving
11 g fat per serving
4 fat units per serving
Preparation time: 35 minutes
Cooking time: 40 minutes

two x 115 g/4 oz chicken paupiettes
or fillets of chicken breast
50 g/2 oz reduced-fat herb and garlic soft cheese
two 25 g/1 oz lean back bacon rashers
2 tsp runny honey

Tarragon dressing:
2 tbsp caster sugar
1 tbsp chopped ginger in syrup, drained
2 tbsp orange juice
2 tbsp lemon juice
1 tbsp fresh tarragon

To serve:
115 g/4 oz apricot coulis
(made from canned apricots, puréed)
2 spring onions
8 cherry tomatoes
4 cm/2 in piece of cucumber
50 g/2 oz yellow pepper
sprinkling of fresh chives, chopped

1 Unravel the paupiettes or flatten the chicken breasts and spread the inside of each with the reduced-fat cheese. Roll up the chicken, wrap a rasher of bacon around the outside and secure with a cocktail stick.

2 Bake in the oven at 180°C/350°F/ gas mark 4 for 35 minutes, until the surface is tinged golden and the bacon becomes crispy. Brush evenly with warm honey.

3 For the tarragon dressing, mix all the dressing ingredients together with a whisk and chill.

4 Serve the chicken warm on the apricot coulis with the sliced salad vegetables and tarragon dressing, sprinkled with fresh chives.

Blueberry-filled baked peaches

SERVES 4

190 calories per serving
2 fat units per serving
6 g fat per serving
Preparation and marinating time: 1½ hours
Cooking time: 30 minutes

4 large ripe peaches or nectarines
3 tbsp brandy
115 ml/4 fl oz unsweetened orange juice
zest of half a lemon
150 g/5 oz blueberries
25 g/10 oz fructose
2 amaretti biscuits, crumbled
2 sponge fingers, crumbled

To Serve:
8 tbsp fromage frais, 8 per cent fat

1 Halve and stone the peaches and place in a non-metallic dish. Sprinkle over the brandy, orange juice and lemon zest and leave to marinate for at least one hour. Meanwhile, heat the blueberries in a non-stick pan until the juices begin to run. Stir in the fructose and cook for a further few minutes.
2 Transfer the peaches to a foil-covered tray. Fill the cavities with some of the blueberries and sprinkle with the biscuit and sponge crumbs and bake at 180°C/350°F/gas mark 4 for 30 minutes.
3 Serve the peaches warm with a spoonful of fromage frais and the remaining blueberries.

Fruit kebabs with mango sauce

SERVES 4

180 calories per serving
½ fat unit equivalent* per serving
0 g fat per serving
Preparation time: 20 minutes
Cooking time: 5 minutes

3 kiwi fruit
8 large strawberries
4 dessert plums, stoned
1 small galia melon
225 g/8 oz large chunks of fresh pineapple
4 level tsp soft brown sugar
pinch of ground cinnamon

Mango sauce:
1 medium ripe mango, stoned
2 tbsp brandy
2 level tbsp honey

1 Peel the kiwi fruit, and cut into bite-sized slices. Halve the strawberries and slice the plums into quarters. Cut the melon in half, remove the seeds, and cut into bite-sized chunks, but don't remove the skin.
2 Thread the fruit onto eight skewers and set to one side. Meanwhile, prepare the mango sauce. Purée the mango in a blender or food processor until smooth. Then stir in the brandy and the honey.

---

* In *Slimming*'s Fat Unit System of dieting (see page 69) a fat unit equivalent value is given to foods which have little or no fat but are high in calories (usually because they are high in sugar) and therefore should be eaten in moderation.

3 Brush the kebabs all over with some of the mango sauce, then sprinkle them with the brown sugar and cinnamon. Grill or barbecue the kebabs until the fruit softens and is tinged golden brown at the edges. This will take between 4 and 5 minutes. Serve two skewers per person with the remaining mango sauce.

Peach mousse

SERVES 6

70 calories per mousse
½ fat unit per mousse
1 g fat per mousse
Preparation and chilling time: 3 hours

1 sachet reduced-sugar orange jelly
225 g/8 oz peaches in natural juice, drained
215 g/7½ oz carton light evaporated milk, chilled

1 Mix the jelly with 275 ml/½ pint boiling water and set to one side to cool. Chill until on the point of setting. Purée the peaches until smooth.
2 Whisk the evaporated milk until it becomes thick and creamy, then fold in the jelly and purée. Mix well and divide evenly between six glasses. Chill until set.

Chocolate fondue

SERVES 2

250 calories per serving
4 fat units per serving
11 g fat per serving
Preparation and chilling time: 1 hour

2 sachets low-calorie milk chocolate drink
115 g/4 oz Greek yogurt
150 g/5 oz fromage frais, 8 per cent fat
175 g/6 oz strawberries
2 kiwi fruit

1 Mix the chocolate drinks with enough boiling water to make a smooth paste. Stir in the yogurt and fromage frais and chill well. Serve half per person in a bowl with sliced strawberries and kiwi fruit, for dipping.

Cherry clafoutis

SERVES 6

170 calories per serving
2 fat units per serving
6 g fat per serving
Preparation and soaking time: 1½ hours
Cooking time: 35–40 minutes

2 tsp oil
450 g/1 lb cherries, pitted
4 tbsp orange juice

3 medium eggs
115 g/4 oz caster sugar
75 g/3 oz plain flour
1 level tbsp icing sugar, to decorate

1 Preheat the oven to 180°C/350°F/gas mark 4. Lightly grease a 1.75 litre/3 pint ovenproof dish with the oil and set to one side. Put the pitted cherries in a bowl, pour the orange juice over them and leave to soak for approximately 1 hour.

2 Place a large, heat-proof bowl over a pan of hot water, then break the eggs into the bowl. Add the sugar and whisk well until the mixture has doubled in size and is pale, thick and creamy.

3 Sieve the plain flour, then fold carefully into the egg mixture.

4 Put the cherries and orange juice in the base of the prepared ovenproof dish, pour the sponge mixture over the top and smooth the surface with a palette knife. Bake for 35 to 40 minutes, or until the sponge is firm to the touch and golden brown. Sprinkle with the icing sugar and serve.

Mixed berries in summer sauce

SERVES 8

150 calories per serving
1 fat unit per serving
2 g fat per serving
Preparation time: 30 minutes
Cooking and chilling time: 1½ hours minimum

275 g/10 oz blackcurrants
225 g/8 oz blueberries
275 g/10 oz redcurrants
350 g/12 oz strawberries, halved or sliced

Sauce:
225 g/8 oz redcurrants
450 g/1 lb raspberries
150 g/5 oz fructose
4 tbsp Kirsch or strawberry liqueur

1 To make the sauce, put the redcurrants, raspberries and fructose in a pan with 3 tbsp water. Heat gently for 10 to 15 minutes, until the juices begin to run. Purée in a blender or food processor until smooth, then cool the purée and stir in the chosen liqueur.

2 Mix the blackcurrants, blueberries and redcurrants with the strawberries and place in a dish. Pour the sauce over the fruit and chill well before serving.

Energy boosters for Autumn

Once the summer weather is over, we tend to pull on baggy sweaters, cut down on the exercising and prepare for hibernation. As the nights get darker and the weather colder, lethargy can set in, and you may risk undoing all the good work you put in getting fit and eating healthily in the summer. However, it's really important to keep your energy levels high in the autumn, to help you feel alert and ward off winter ailments like colds and flu.

Try these energy-packed recipes for main meals, snacks and drinks, to help you lose weight and keep you on tip-top form.

Pork medallions with cider sauce

SERVES 2

395 calories per serving
5 fat units per serving
14 g fat per serving
Preparation time: 15 minutes
Cooking time: 40 minutes

4 level tsp plain flour
salt and freshly ground black pepper
pinch of dried sage
four 50 g/2 oz lean pork medallions
4 tsp oil
1 small red onion, finely chopped
6 garlic cloves, trimmed
2 tsp wholegrain mustard
1 medium apple, cored and sliced
1 medium pear, cored and sliced
50 ml/2 fl oz fresh chicken stock
150 ml/¼ pint dry cider
4 rosemary sprigs

1 Season the flour with the salt and dried sage, then use to coat the pork evenly.
2 Heat half the oil in a non-stick pan and sauté the onion for 4 to 5 minutes until softened. Add the garlic cloves and cook for a few minutes until they begin to turn golden at the edges.
3 Add the remaining oil and the pork and cook for 4 to 5 minutes on each side, until it loses its pinky colour and the edges are tinged golden brown.
4 Meanwhile, cook the apple and pear slices in the chicken stock for 5 minutes until tender. Strain, reserving the stock, and set the fruit to one side.

5 Add the mustard, cider, chicken stock and rosemary sprigs to the pork and bring to the boil. Reduce the heat and simmer for 20 minutes until the sauce has reduced and thickened.

6 Add the fruit to the pan and heat through. Season to taste and serve at once.

Stuffed tomatoes

SERVES 2

350 calories per serving
5 fat units per serving
16 g fat per serving
Preparation time: 25 minutes
Cooking time: 30 minutes

four 175 g/6 oz beef tomatoes
75 g/3 oz lean back bacon rashers, well grilled
2 tsp oil
2 spring onions, roughly chopped
1 small yellow pepper, deseeded and diced
175 g/6 oz instant rice, canned or frozen
2 level tsp sun-dried tomato paste
freshly ground black pepper
25 g/1 oz reduced-fat mature Cheddar cheese
fresh parsley, chopped, to garnish
lettuce and cherry tomatoes, to serve

1 Preheat the oven to 180°C/350°F/gas mark 4. Slice off the tops of the beef tomatoes and remove some flesh. Discard the seeds and juice and roughly chop the removed tomato flesh. Place the tomato shells in an oven-proof dish.

2 Cut the well-grilled bacon into bite-sized pieces.

3 Heat the oil in a non-stick pan and sauté the onions and pepper for 3 to 4 minutes until softened. Stir in the rice, chopped tomato and bacon and cook for a further 2 minutes.

4 Stir in the tomato paste and mix well. Season with freshly ground black pepper.

5 Fill the tomatoes with the mixture, sprinkle with cheese and bake for 20 minutes, until the tomatoes are tender and the cheese has turned golden brown. Garnish with parsley and serve with lettuce and cherry tomatoes.

Gingered beef stir-fry

SERVES 2

310 calories per serving
5 fat units per serving
14 g fat per serving
Preparation time: 15 minutes
Cooking time: 15 minutes

225 g/8 oz lean beef or sirloin steak
2 tbsp Teriyaki sauce
3 tbsp unsweetened orange juice
sprinkling of ground ginger
2 tbsp dry sherry
1 level tsp cornflour
4 tsp oil
1 small red onion, sliced
1 small yellow pepper, deseeded and sliced
75 g/3 oz button mushrooms, halved
75 g/3 oz mangetout peas
50 g/2 oz baby corn, halved

1 Cut the beef into thin strips.
2 Mix the Teriyaki sauce in a bowl with the orange juice, ground ginger and sherry and stir in the cornflour until well blended.
3 Heat the oil for a few minutes in a non-stick frying-pan, then add the beef and cook for 3 to 4 minutes, stirring occasionally. Add vegetables and stir-fry until the vegetables are cooked.
4 Pour the sauce into the pan and mix until it thickens and has coated the meat and vegetables evenly.

Tuna potato layer

SERVES 4

350 calories per serving
5 fat units per serving
14 g fat per serving
Preparation time: 25 minutes
Cooking time: 40 minutes

350 g/12 oz potatoes, (peeled weight), thinly sliced
two 200 g/7 oz cans tuna in brine, drained
pinch of dried herbes de Provence
2 tomatoes, sliced
115 g/4 oz leeks, sliced
525 g/18½ oz carton lasagne sauce for tuna
75 g/3 oz reduced-fat mature Cheddar cheese, grated
sliced tomato and lettuce, to serve

1 Preheat the oven to 190°C/375°F/gas mark 5. Simmer the potatoes in lightly salted water for 10 minutes. Drain well and set aside.

2 Break the tuna into bite-sized chunks and mix with the herbes de Provence.

3 Place a layer of potatoes in the base of an ovenproof dish, cover with a layer of tuna followed by a layer of tomatoes and then one of leeks. Repeat the layers. Pour the tuna sauce over the dish, then sprinkle with cheese.

4 Bake for 25 minutes, until the topping has become crispy. Serve with the lettuce and tomato.

Pitta pockets

MAKES 1 PITTA POCKET

150 calories per pocket
1½ fat units per pocket
4 g fat per pocket
Preparation time: 5 minutes

3 cherry tomatoes, halved
quarter of a small red onion, finely chopped
lettuce, shredded
40 g/1½ oz reduced-calorie coleslaw
35 g/1¼ oz canned mixed beans, drained
1 mini pitta bread

1 Mix the tomatoes, onion and some lettuce with the coleslaw and beans. Chill until required. Fill the pitta pocket with the salad and serve with extra lettuce.

Chicken and bean bread pot

SERVES 4

360 calories per serving
3 fat units per serving
8 g fat per serving
Preparation time: 20 minutes
Cooking time: 20 minutes

a 450 g/1 lb white loaf of bread
400 g/14 oz can baked beans and frankfurters
in tomato sauce
1 medium onion, sliced
1 green and 1 red pepper, medium-sized,
deseeded and sliced
225 g/8 oz lean cooked chicken, diced

1 Preheat the oven to 180°C/350°F/gas mark 4. Slice the top off the loaf and scoop out the centre, leaving a 2.5 cm/½ inch border. Keep crumbs for another dish that requires breadcrumbs.

2 Thoroughly heat the beans with the onion, peppers and chicken. Spoon this mixture into the hollow loaf and warm in the oven. Serve at once with a green salad.

Mixed berry brulées

MAKES 8 BRULÉES

205 calories per brulée
3½ fat units per brulée
10 g fat per brulée
Preparation time: 25 minutes, plus chilling
Cooking time: 1 hour

450 g/1 lb reduced-fat crème fraîche
175 g/6 oz fat-free fromage frais
1 vanilla pod
3 medium egg yolks
pinch of dried cinnamon
115 g/4 oz caster sugar

To decorate:
3 dessert plums, stoned and sliced
75 g/3 oz raspberries
75 g/3 oz blackberries

1 Heat the crème fraîche and vanilla pod together until almost boiling, then leave to infuse for at least an hour. Then remove the vanilla pod and stir in the fromage frais.

2 Preheat the oven to 150 °C/300 °F/gas mark 2. Beat together the egg yolks, cinnamon and 50 g/2 oz of the sugar until the mixture is light and creamy in colour. Gradually pour on the crème fraîche, stirring until evenly mixed, to create a custard.

3 Stand six individual ramekin dishes in a roasting dish containing enough hot water to reach half-way up the sides of the ramekins. Pour the custard slowly into the ramekins, dividing it equally between them.

4 Bake in the oven for about 1 hour, until the custard is set but without allowing the skin to colour. Remove the ramekins from the tin and leave to cool. Chill overnight in the fridge.

5 Sprinkle the remaining sugar evenly over each brulée, then place under a medium-hot grill until the sugar caramelizes. Allow to cool, then decorate each brulée with the fruit and serve.

Autumn muffins

MAKES 12 MUFFINS

150 calories per muffin
1½ fat units per muffin
2 g fat per muffin
Preparation time: 25 minutes
Cooking time: 20 minutes

1 medium pear, chopped
275 g/10 oz plain flour
pinch of salt
2 level tsp baking powder
½ tsp ground mixed spice
75 g/3 oz fructose
2 medium eggs
150 ml/¼ pt semi-skimmed milk
50 g/2 oz half-fat spread, melted
75 g/3 oz blackberries or raspberries

1 Cook the pear until tender and, set to one side. Preheat the oven to 180°C/350°F/gas mark 4. Line twelve bun tins with paper cases.
2 Sieve the flour into a large mixing bowl with the salt, baking powder and mixed spice. Stir in the fructose.
3 In another bowl, lightly beat together the eggs, milk and melted spread, then add to the pear and fruit mixture and mix together roughly. Add the flour and stir until evenly distributed.
4 Spoon the mixture into the paper cases and bake in the centre of the oven for 20 minutes until golden brown and firm to the touch.

Flapjacks

MAKES 12 FLAPJACKS

150 calories per flapjack
2 fat units per flapjack
6 g fat per flapjack
Preparation time: 10 minutes
Cooking time: 25 minutes

75 g/3 oz ready to eat dried apricots, roughly chopped
75 g/3 oz ready to eat dried dates, roughly chopped
pinch of ground cinnamon
200 g/7 oz porridge oats
25 g/1 oz soft brown sugar
115 g/4 oz low-fat spread
4 level tbsp runny honey
1 level tsp icing sugar, to decorate

1 Line a square, shallow 18 cm/7 inch baking tin with non-stick baking paper. Preheat the oven to 180 °C/350 °F/gas mark 4.
2 Put the apricots and dates in a bowl with the cinnamon, porridge oats and sugar. Melt the low-fat spread with the honey until the mixture is runny. Stir into the oats mixture and mix well.
3 Transfer to the baking tin and level the surface with a palette knife. Bake for 20 to 25 minutes, until golden and firm to the touch. Cool for 5 minutes before turning out, then cut into twelve equal squares. Sprinkle with icing sugar before serving.

Fruit cocktail

MAKES 2 COCKTAILS

150 calories per cocktail
0 fat units per cocktail
0 g fat per cocktail
Preparation time: 10 minutes

1 medium apple
1 small orange
115 g/4 oz grapes
175 g/6 oz galia melon, skinned
115 g/4 oz raspberries
175 g/6 oz fresh pineapple in natural juice
artificial sweetener, to taste

1 Cut the fruit into bite-sized chunks and mix together.
Add the sweetener and chill until required.

Banana shake

MAKES 4 DRINKS

150 calories per drink
1 fat units per drink
3 g fat per drink
Preparation time: 5 minutes

2 medium bananas
1 level tbsp soft brown sugar
1 tbsp lemon juice
425 ml/¾ pint skimmed milk
75 g/3 oz carton low-fat Greek yogurt with honey
mint sprigs, to serve (optional)

1 Mash the bananas, sugar and lemon juice together with a fork until smooth. Place the mixture in a blender with the milk and yogurt and process until smooth. Chill until required, then serve garnished with mint, if liked.

Mixed berry shake

MAKES 2 DRINKS

150 calories per drink
3 fat units per drink
9 g fat per drink
Preparation time: 5 minutes

150 g/5 oz raspberries
350 ml/12 fl oz skimmed milk
200 g/7 oz carton strawberry-flavoured diet fromage frais,
8 per cent fat
1 level tbsp caster sugar

1 Put the raspberries, milk and fromage frais in a blender and process until smooth. Sweeten with sugar and serve.

Warming wonders for Winter

Winter diet tips

- A saucepan of soup simmering on the stove could be just the thing to cheer you up on a cold day. Make up a huge pan of soup with some low-calorie vegetables, water, stock cubes and herbs. Keep a soup supply in the fridge (or in the freezer, if you make enough), then reheat portions whenever you wish. The soup is so low in calories and fat you'll be able to fill up on it easily without ruining your diet.

- Make sure you include plenty of fresh fruit in your diet, especially oranges and grapefruit. Although the debate about whether vitamin C can prevent colds continues, it can do no harm to feast on fruit and it could do your diet some good.

- Beware of pigging out when you switch from summer dresses to cover-all chunky sweaters. It's easy to pretend that a weight problem doesn't exist when you hide it away. Wear something with a fitted waistband at least once a week to give you a warning of any waistline expansion.

- There's no need to fill up on stodge just because it's cold. A baked potato with a low-calorie topping makes a warming and filling lunch. You can even afford to eat rice pudding if you make it with skimmed milk and stir in some sweetener.

- Does a switch from cold drinks to hot usually mean your liquid consumption dives in winter? It is important, especially if your diet includes lots of fibre, to have plenty of low-calorie liquids. A warm drink can help you relax and stop you from nibbling, too. Tea served with lemon, black coffee and herbal tea are all calorie-free; Bovril and Marmite contain about 10 calories a cup, and a low-calorie hot chocolate drink around 35–40 calories.

- Losing a layer of fat may make you feel the cold more, but eating fat won't make you feel warmer again (except by helping you put that layer of fat back on). Only explorers sledging through icy wastes can get away with eating a diet high in fat. That's because they can expend up to 5000 calories a day. Low-fat meals that add up to this amount of calories would be just too bulky to swallow – another reason why reducing your fat intake helps you lose weight.

- Prepare for a party by cutting down on calories a few days beforehand to save them up. Take the edge off your appetite before you go by eating a piece of fruit, a low-fat chocolate bar or a small can of reduced-sugar baked beans on a piece of toast.

- If you do over-indulge at a party, work out a menu that you can follow the next day to undo the damage. If you are slimming on 1500 calories a day, cut down to 1000. But if your daily allowance is 1000 calories, don't be tempted to drop below 700 calories – and definitely for no longer than a day. Rather than risk getting caught in a starve-binge cycle, it's better to put your over-indulgence down to experience and postpone your target-weight date slightly.

- If you buy chocolates, cakes and edible Christmas goodies early, you may find they start calling 'Eat me!' from the cupboard! Buy non-food Christmas things first and leave the food as late as you can to minimize this risk.

- Sipping a hot toddy may warm you up initially, but alcohol will eventually make you feel colder (and don't forget the damage it may inflict on your diet).

- Don't let bad weather put you off exercising if your favourite outdoor sports are impossible. Look around for indoor alternatives or exercise at home with a video or by indoor mountaineering (climbing up and down stairs!).

- Make sure you make the most of the limited winter daylight. A brisk walk every day can ward off the winter gloom and helps you feel more alert. If dark days always make you very down and lethargic, you may have SAD (Seasonal Affective Disorder). Effective treatments are available (see your GP for advice).

The following substantial main-course recipes all provide 400 calories or less per portion and are low in fat, too. Serve them with a large portion of steamed or boiled green vegetables to complete a filling, warming meal.

Cheese and onion potato pie

SERVES 4

295 calories per serving
3½ fat units per serving
10 g fat per serving
Preparation time: 30 minutes
Cooking time: 35 minutes

575 g/1½ lb potatoes (peeled weight)
115 g/4 oz onion
2 tsp oil
75 g/3 oz reduced-fat Cheddar cheese
425 ml/¾ pint semi-skimmed milk
25 g/1 oz half-fat spread
25 g/1 oz plain flour
half a level tsp dry mustard
salt and freshly ground black pepper
sprigs of parsley and chopped parsley, to garnish

1 Preheat the oven to 200 °C/400 °F/gas mark 6. Slice the potatoes, then add them to a pan of boiling water and cook for 5 minutes. Drain.
2 Thinly slice the onion. Heat the oil in a non-stick pan and fry the onion until soft and golden. Grate the cheese.
3 Put the milk, half-fat spread and flour in a pan and bring to the boil, whisking continuously. Add the mustard and three-quarters of the cheese. Season with salt and pepper.

4 Layer the potatoes and onions in an ovenproof dish. Then pour the sauce over them and sprinkle with the remaining cheese. Bake for 30 to 35 minutes. Garnish with parsley and serve.

Honey-glazed chicken

SERVES 4

360 calories per serving
3½ fat units per serving
10 g fat per serving
Preparation time: 10 minutes
Cooking time: 1 hour

four 150 g/5 oz chicken breasts, skinned
2 level tbsp honey
freshly ground black pepper
175 g/6 oz button mushrooms
400 g/14 oz can apricots in natural juice
425 ml/¾ pint ready-made white wine sauce
2 tbsp fresh parsley, chopped, to garnish

1 Preheat the oven to 190 °C/375 °F/gas mark 5. Place the chicken breasts in an ovenproof dish. Brush with honey and sprinkle with pepper.
2 Slice the mushrooms and drain and halve the apricots. Add the mushrooms, apricots and wine sauce to the chicken.
3 Bake in the oven for 1 hour, until the chicken is tender and cooked through. Garnish with parsley before serving.

Steak and kidney pie

SERVES 4

405 calories per serving
5 fat units per serving
14 g fat per serving
Preparation time: 40 minutes, plus 1 hour cooling time
Cooking time: 3 hours

350 g/12 oz lean braising beef
115 g/4 oz lamb's kidneys
150 g/5 oz plain flour, plus 3 level tbsp flour
salt and freshly ground black pepper
75 g/3 oz button mushrooms
50 g/2 oz carrots
75g/3oz onion
1 beef stock cube
275 ml/½ pint beer
65 g/2½ oz half-fat spread
1 small egg

1 Preheat the oven to 150 °C/300 °F/gas mark 2. Cut the beef into small pieces. Halve the kidneys, discard the white cores, and cut into small pieces. Season 2 level tbsp flour. Toss the beef and the kidney in the seasoned flour and place in a casserole dish.

2 Halve the mushrooms, slice the carrots and chop the onion. Add to the meat and crumble the stock cube on top. Pour in the beer. Cover and cook in the oven for 2½ hours. Turn into a pie dish and leave to cool. Increase the oven temperature to 190 °C/375 °F/gas mark 5.

3 Rub the half-fat spread into 150 g/5 oz of the flour. Lightly beat the egg and stir half of it into the flour. Add enough cold water to make a stiff dough. Roll out using

the remaining tablespoon of flour and place on the meat. Brush with the remaining egg and bake for 20 to 30 minutes, until brown on top.

Chicken and leek pie

SERVES 4

365 calories per serving
4½ fat units per serving
13 g fat per serving
Preparation time: 30 minutes
Cooking time: 50 minutes

2 rashers extra-lean back bacon
275 g/10 oz cooked chicken, skinned
4 baby leeks
75 g/3 oz carrots
425 g/15 oz white wine cooking sauce
salt and freshly ground black pepper
575 g/1¼ lb potatoes (peeled weight)
25 g/1 oz half-fat spread
4 tbsp semi-skimmed milk
sprigs of parsley, to garnish

1 Preheat the oven to 190 °C/375 °F/gas mark 5. Grill the bacon and cut into small pieces. Cut the chicken into small pieces and trim and slice the leeks. Place the bacon, chicken and leeks in an ovenproof dish.
2 Slice the carrots, boil for 10 minutes and drain. Add to the chicken dish with the sauce. Season to taste.
3 Boil the potatoes. Drain well and mash with the spread and the milk. Pipe or spread on top of the chicken and bake for 25 to 30 minutes. Garnish with parsley.

Pork and apple with dumplings

SERVES 4

335 calories per serving
5½ fat units per serving
16 g fat per serving
Preparation time: 20 minutes
Cooking time: 45 minutes

450 g/1 lb lean boneless pork chump steak
1 chicken stock cube
1 small red or yellow pepper
4 baby leeks
50 g/2 oz button mushrooms
50 g/2 oz self-raising flour
25 g/1 oz shredded suet
1 tsp fresh sage, chopped,
or half a level tsp dried sage
1 tsp fresh parsley, chopped,
plus sprigs of parsley to garnish
25 g/1 oz breadcrumbs
salt and freshly ground pepper
1 medium eating apple, Cox's or Granny Smith's
1 level tbsp cornflour
4 tbsp reduced-fat crème fraîche
1 level tbsp grainy French mustard

1 Cut the pork into small pieces and cook in a non-stick pan until it changes colour. Add 350 ml/12 fl oz water and the stock cube (dissolved in 3 tbsp water), cover and simmer for 15 minutes. Cut the deseeded pepper into small pieces, slice the leeks and halve the mushrooms. Add them to the pork. Cover and simmer for 5 minutes.

2 Meanwhile, mix together the flour, suet, herbs, bread-crumbs, seasoning and 3 tbsp water to make a firm dough. Shape into eight balls. Add to the pan, cover and cook for 15 minutes. Core the apple and cut into large pieces. Add to the pan and cook for a further 5 minutes.

3 Remove the meat, apples, vegetables and dumplings from the pan and set aside. Mix together the cornflour, crème fraîche and mustard. Add to the pan and mix well. Simmer for 1 minute, whisking gently all the time. Return the meat and dumplings to the pan and heat through. Garnish with parsley.

Chicken and pasta bake

SERVES 4

395 calories per serving
3½ fat units per serving
10 g fat per serving
Preparation time: 15 minutes
Cooking time: 1 hour 10 minutes

115 g/4 oz pasta shapes (dry weight)
four 150 g/5 oz chicken breasts, skinned
150 g/5 oz button mushrooms
1 tsp mixed dried herbs
115 g/4 oz bottled mixed peppers in tomato dressing
295 g can condensed half-fat chicken soup
freshly ground black pepper
50 g/2 oz reduced-fat Cheddar cheese, grated
fresh parsley, to garnish

1 Preheat the oven to 190 °C/375 °F/gas mark 5. Boil the pasta until tender, then transfer to an ovenproof dish. Cut the chicken into bite-sized pieces and slice the mushrooms. Add the chicken, mushrooms and herbs to the pasta.

2 Add the peppers, soup and a can of cold water, then toss the mixture to coat the pasta evenly. Season.

3 Sprinkle with cheese and bake in the oven for 1 hour, until golden brown. Garnish with the parsley.

Old-fashioned rice pudding

SERVES 6

155 calories per serving
1½ fat units per serving
4 g fat per serving
Preparation time: 20 minutes
Cooking time: 3 hours

1 tsp oil
50 g/2 oz pudding rice
2 tsp caster sugar
850 ml/1½ pints semi-skimmed milk
1 bay-leaf
freshly grated nutmeg
2 oranges
25 g/1 oz half-fat spread
1 tsp icing sugar

1 Preheat the oven to 170 °C/325 °F/gas mark 3. Lightly grease a shallow, ovenproof 1.7 litre/3 pint dish. Add the rice, sugar, milk, bay-leaf and nutmeg and stir gently.

2 Stir in the zest and juice of one orange. Dot the pudding with knobs of the half-fat spread, then stand the dish on a baking tray and bake for 30 minutes.

3 Remove from oven and stir. Return to the oven for a further 2 hours (covering with foil after 1 hour) or until most of the milk is absorbed and a golden-brown skin has formed.

4 Sprinkle with nutmeg and icing sugar, decorate with a few reserved orange slices and serve.

Apple Charlotte

SERVES 8

210 calories per serving
1 fat unit per serving
3 g fat per serving
Preparation time: 30 minutes
Cooking time: 40 minutes

565 g/1¼ lb stewed apples
75 g/30 oz fructose
sprinkling of ground cinnamon or ginger
50 g/2 oz half-fat spread, softened
200 g/7 oz white medium-sliced bread
(weight with crusts removed)
3 tbsp honey

To serve:
1 medium orange, sliced
350 g/12 oz reduced-fat, ready to serve custard

1 Preheat the oven to 180 °C/350 °F/gas mark 4. Mix the apple with the fructose and cinnamon or ginger.

2 Use a little of the half-fat spread to grease a 1.4 litre/
  2½ pt pudding basin and line the base with greaseproof
  paper.
3 Cover one side of each slice of bread with the remaining
  spread, then use three-quarters of the slices to line the
  base and sides of the basin, with the spread side facing
  outwards.
4 Spoon in the stewed-apple purée and cover with the
  remaining bread, spread facing outwards, to seal in the
  purée. Bake for 35 to 40 minutes, until the bread is
  golden brown and firm to the touch.
5 Brush with honey and serve topped with orange slices
  and a jug of hot custard.

Banana bake

SERVES 4

280 calories per serving
1 fat unit per serving
3 g fat per serving
Preparation time: 15 minutes
Cooking time: 30 minutes

275 g/10 oz fresh pineapple or canned pineapple
in natural juice (flesh only)
411 g/14½ oz can apricot halves in natural juice
2 large bananas, thickly sliced
4 slices white bread
2 level tbsp half-fat spread
2 tbsp honey

1 Cube the pineapple and place in a casserole dish with the
  apricots and their juice and the sliced bananas.

2 Spread the bread with the half-fat spread and honey. Cut into triangles and arrange on top of the fruit.
3 Bake at 190 °C/375 °F/gas mark 5 for 20 to 30 minutes, or until the top is golden.

Gingernut crumble

SERVES 6

245 calories per serving
2 fat units per serving
7 g fat per serving
Preparation time: 20 minutes
Cooking time: 1 hour 10 minutes

411 g/14½ oz can pears in juice
4 trifle sponges
4 level tsp ginger marmalade
4 medium eggs
425 ml/5 fl oz semi-skimmed milk
50 g/2 oz fructose
few drops vanilla essence
6 reduced-fat gingernut biscuits, crushed

1 Drain the pears, reserving 4 tbsp of the juice. Halve the sponges lengthways, spread with marmalade and sandwich together. Place in a dish, with the pears. Sprinkle with the reserved pear juice.
2 Beat together the eggs, milk and fructose using a hand whisk. Add the vanilla essence. Pour the mixture onto the sponges.
3 Bake at 180 °C/350 °F/gas mark 4 for 1 hour 10 minutes, or until lightly set. Top with the crushed gingernut biscuits and serve.

Eve's pudding

SERVES 6

150 calories per serving
1 fat unit per serving
2 g fat per serving
Preparation time: 30 minutes
Cooking time: 25 minutes

675 g/1½ lb eating apples
(e.g. Cox's, Granny Smith's)
3 tbsp apple juice
2 medium eggs
65 g/1½ oz caster sugar
50 g/2 oz plain flour

1 Peel and core the apples. Slice and cook in a covered pan with the apple juice until tender. Divide the mixture between six small ovenproof dishes.
2 Preheat the oven to 180 °C/350 °F/gas mark 4. Put the eggs and sugar in a large bowl placed over a pan of simmering water, and whisk until pale and creamy. The mixture should be thick enough to leave a trail on the surface when the whisk is lifted out.
3 Sieve the flour into the bowl and gently fold into the mixture. Divide between the small dishes and bake for 15 minutes.

Scotch pancakes

MAKES 14 PANCAKES

80 calories per topped pancake
1 fat unit per topped pancake
3 g fat per topped pancake
Preparation time: 10 minutes
Cooking time: 35 minutes

oil for greasing
115 g/4 oz self-raising flour
2 level tbsp caster sugar
zest of 1 lemon
zest of 1 orange
1 large egg, beaten
150 ml/¼ pint semi-skimmed milk
6 level tbsp reduced-sugar jam
6 level tbsp reduced-fat crème fraîche

1 Lightly grease and preheat a griddle or large non-stick frying pan.
2 Mix the flour and caster sugar in a large bowl with the lemon and orange zest. Make a well in the centre and stir in the eggs and milk to make a batter the consistency of thick cream.
3 Drop the mixture in spoonfuls on to the hot griddle or frying-pan. After 2 to 3 minutes bubbles will rise to the surface; when this happens, turn the pancakes over.
4 Cook for a further 2 to 3 minutes until golden brown, then remove and allow to cool while you cook the rest of the pancakes. Serve topped with the jam and crème fraîche.

5

Strategies for a fitter body

Why exercise matters

Many people's image of physical activity is pain and strain.
Avoid being forced into an exercise routine that you dislike,
and which makes you feel anything less than energized. The
right sort of exercise is enjoyable, and can give your energy
levels a real boost.

When you exercise, your body produces chemicals
called endorphins, which are well known for their 'feel-
good' effect. It's never too late to start exercising. In fact,
the older you are, the more important it is to keep your
body supple. Exercise can improve the quality of your life
and health. The important thing is to find the right kind of
exercise to suit you, your lifestyle and your fitness level.

There are plenty of good reasons why you should take
exercise: for example, it strengthens immunity, reduces the
risk of brittle bone disease (osteoporosis) and improves cir-
culation; the enhanced flow of oxygen to the cells helps
keep blood pressure and cholesterol levels normal. Exercise
can also improve mental health. And those are just a few of
the beneficial effects.

Regular exercise can increase the proportion of lean
muscle tissue you have in your body. Lean tissue needs
more energy to sustain it than fat tissue, so the more lean

tissue you have in your body, the more calories your body burns up, even if you're just sitting around. Increasing your resting metabolic rate through exercise will help you get slim and stay slim.

Consider every type of exercise before you make a decision about which will suit you best. If nothing else, brisk walking for half an hour each day should keep you in shape and feeling energized, providing you're not breathing in fumes and battling with articulated lorries.

If you are really not used to physical activity, start off with some simple stretching exercises like those shown later in this chapter, and gradually increase your routine until you are doing a minimum of three 20-minute exercise routines every week.

If you're always on the go – running around after children, shopping and so on – you'll be getting plenty of exercise and burning off calories. But sometimes this isn't enough. To get the full benefits from exercise, you may need to take some aerobic form of activity (the sort that makes you feel slightly breathless over a sustained period).

Fitness plan for suppleness, strength and stamina

There's a lot of confusing jargon about getting fit, but basically all you need to remember are the three s's: suppleness, strength and stamina. These are the three essential elements of being fit, and to achieve all-round fitness you need to take different kinds of regular exercise that will improve all three of them.

Some activities may be easy for you, others more difficult, depending on a number of factors, such as how active you currently are, and your natural body make-up. For instance, some people can easily touch their toes but would find it hard to walk briskly for 20 minutes; others may be able to play tennis for an hour but couldn't lift a heavy piece of furniture. What's important is that you have a healthy balance of varied activities, which will help improve your suppleness, strength and stamina.

Below are some suggestions to help you get working on these three key fitness areas. They have been devised by Jon LeBon, a fitness expert and personal trainer who is himself a successful slimmer. Having been overweight all his life, he lost an amazing 15 stone (96 kilos) nearly ten years ago, slimming from 29 stone (184 kilos) to a healthy 13 stone 12 (88 kilos). Still slim and super-fit, he specializes in helping overweight clients achieve their fitness goals.

Suppleness

This means being able to bend, stretch, twist and turn with ease. It means being able to reach for a tin on a high shelf, get in and out of the car without strain and bend down to tie up your shoelaces in comfort. Being supple reduces the risk of being injured, helps you stay active as you get older and makes you look and feel much younger.

Jon LeBon's stretch plan

Make these stretches part of your daily schedule. They are particularly valuable when done as a sequence straight after a session of stamina-building activity. Always move slowly and smoothly into a stretch and then hold. Don't bounce.

Upper back stretch
Imagine you are hugging a large ball with your arms out and palms slightly overlapped. Move your shoulders and arms forward and hold still for a count of eight. You should feel a stretch in your upper back.

Shoulder and chest stretch
Reach your arms behind you with your elbows bent. Draw your shoulders back and hold for a count of eight.

Triceps stretch
Place your left arm across your chest at shoulder height. Hold on to the back of your upper left arm with your right hand. Use your right hand to ease your left arm further across the front of your body and then hold for a count of eight. Repeat with your right arm.

Full body stretch
Lie on your back. Extend your arms and legs away from your body along the floor and stretch them without lifting them off the floor. Hold for a count of twelve. You should be able to feel your whole body stretching.

Hamstring stretch
Lie on your back with your knees bent so the soles of your feet are on the floor. Slowly lift and straighten your left leg, bringing it towards your head. When you start to feel the stretch down the back of your leg, hold for a count of twelve. Repeat with your right leg.

Gluteal (bottom) stretch
In a sitting position, cross your left leg over your right leg. Then lean forwards, bringing your right shoulder across to your left knee and gently hug your left knee with both arms. Hold for a count of twelve. Repeat with your right knee and left shoulder.

Adductor stretch
In a sitting position, and with your knees bent, bring the soles of your feet together and, with a straight back, lean forwards slowly. Hold for a count of twelve.

Strength

This doesn't mean bulging muscles, but the ability to carry your toddler, climb stairs and push the mower over the lawn. Working to strengthen or tone your muscles will protect you from sprains and strains and help improve the look and shape of your outline. Strong muscles in your back will also improve your posture. Good toning activities include swimming, cycling, weight training and digging.

Jon LeBon's tone plan

These exercises are designed to give all-over body strength. As you get stronger you will be able to do more repetitions of each exercise. To start with, try eight repetitions, but if this is too difficult, just do as many as you can. Try to add one or two more repetitions each week.

Chest, shoulders and back of upper arms

Put your palms against a wall at shoulder height. Slightly bend your knees to lower your body and lean it in towards the wall. Now use your arms to push your body back from the wall, squeezing your arms and chest muscles as you push the weight of your body back.

Shoulders

Stand with your feet hip width apart and your arms hanging by your side. Slowly raise your arms to shoulder height, with your elbows very slightly bent and palms down. Imagine that you are pushing up against some form of resistance.

Buttocks and legs

Rest one hand on the back of a chair for balance. Take a step forwards with one foot and slowly drop your back knee to the floor with a lungeing action. Now gently rise up to a standing position again and repeat on the other side.

Front of upper arm
Stand with your hands by your sides, palms upwards. With your pelvis slightly tilted forwards and knees a little bent, slowly curl your lower arm up towards your shoulders. As you bring your arm up, imagine that you are pushing against a heavy weight.

Tummy
Lie on your back with your hands resting on your thighs. Gently raise your shoulders off the floor, hold for a count of two and then slowly relax.

Lower back
Lie on your front with your arms by your sides. Gently raise your shoulders off the floor, hold for a count of two and then slowly relax.

Stamina

This means being able to keep going for a long time at a good pace, whether you're walking, running, cycling, or simply going about everyday tasks. If you have plenty of stamina you will be able to rush to get to the office on time, give the windows a good clean without getting puffed out, and enjoy going swimming with the kids.

Activities for building stamina are known as 'aerobic' because the intensity of the exercise makes you breathe in a lot of oxygen to supply your hard-working muscles. This kind of activity increases the efficiency of your heart and lungs and helps burn fat. Any activity that raises your heart rate and makes you feel slightly out of breath will improve stamina.

It is important to warm up before aerobic exercise with gentle bends and stretches and to cool down afterwards by walking for a few minutes or doing more stretches.

Jon LeBon's stamina programme
Vary these activities as much as possible to keep boredom at bay. Choose from:

brisk walking	gardening
circuit training	jogging
cycling	netball
aerobics	running
badminton	stair-climbing
dancing	swimming energetically
fitness class	tennis
football	vigorous housework

Jon LeBon's top ten fitness tips

1 Exercise is for everyone. Whatever your age, level of fitness, natural skill or size, there's something out there for you. It's just a question of doing your research to find an activity that suits you.

2 If you're not used to exercising, start gradually and slowly increase your level of activity. You'll be amazed at how quickly and easily you start to feel an improvement.

3 Exercise doesn't have to hurt to be doing you good – quite the reverse. Try chanting the nursery rhyme 'Mary had a little lamb' while you exercise. If you can sing it easily, you need to push yourself harder; if you're too puffed to get the words out, then slow down a little.

4 Enter your activity sessions in your diary. If you set a particular time aside, you will be more likely to keep your appointment with yourself. Once you start exercising you'll find it becomes a habit that fits easily into your life.

5 Try to be more active in your everyday life. Take the stairs instead of the lift, push the vacuum cleaner with a bit more gusto and try to walk or cycle rather than taking the car on short journeys. Small changes can make a big difference.

6 Set yourself challenges to keep up your interest. Aim to walk the same distance in less time or enrol in another kind of exercise class.

7 It's important that you enjoy exercise. Some people prefer the discipline of a class, others prefer to be on their own, some like to be competitive, others want to exercise for fun. We're all different, so don't give up at the first hurdle. Experiment until you find what's right for you.

8 Exercising with a friend can give you the support you need. Encourage your nearest and dearest to join you.

9 Keep a record of how much better you feel. Note the changes in your sense of well-being and your body shape. This will act as a reminder of why you want to keep active.

10 Make a commitment to exercise. You can't store fitness – it must be a regular part of your life.

Index

Slim and save money with
SLIMMING MAGAZINE CLUBS

Having moral support from people who understand exactly how you feel can make all the difference to a successful slimming campaign. Every year, thousands of successful slimmers find that Slimming Magazine Clubs are just the place to find all the expert, friendly help and support they need.

Slimming Magazine Clubs are one of the country's top slimming organizations, and they have hundreds of clubs throughout England, Wales and Scotland. All Slimming Magazine Club group leaders are specially trained and – just as importantly – they have all conquered a weight problem themselves. Who better to understand the needs and concerns of slimmers?

Slimming Magazine Club meetings are friendly and fun. They're confidential too; your weight remains a secret between you and your group leader – at least until you've reached target and want to tell the world about it! A typical meeting will include a group discussion and project; an inspirational, informative talk from your group leader, and time to chat and swap tips and stories with fellow slimmers.

You can sit through a meeting before deciding to join. If you do, your group leader will discuss your diet problems with you and recommend one of Slimming Magazine Clubs' wide range of healthy-eating diets, designed to cater for all types of slimmer from vegans to chocoholics! After that she'll monitor your progress carefully week by week and will always be happy to offer advice and support.

As a special invitation to *Dare To Bare* readers, Slimming Magazine Clubs are offering FREE membership – saving you £6.00.

All you have to do is take the voucher overleaf along to your nearest club.

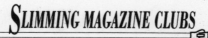

SLIMMING MAGAZINE CLUBS